SLEEP
POSITIONS

SLEEP POSITIONS

The Night Language of the Body

by SAMUEL DUNKELL, *M.D.*

WILLIAM MORROW AND COMPANY, INC.
NEW YORK   1977

Drawings by Ruth Dunkell

Printed in the United States of America.

1   2   3   4   5   6   7   8   9   10

Library of Congress Cataloging in Publication Data

Dunkell, Samuel.
    Sleep positions.

    1. Sleep positions. I. Title.
BF1073.S56D86   154.6   76-42243
ISBN 0-688-03152-8

BOOK DESIGN   CARL WEISS

FOR
RUTH AND LIZ

CONTENTS

PREFACE

I FIRST BECAME AWARE that sleep positions had special significance some years ago, during a psychotherapy session with a
young female patient. Discussing her difficulty in establishing
good relationships with men, she told me that the position
in which she slept contributed to her problem. She slept
facedown, she said, with her arms and legs spread out, encompassing as much of the bed as she could. Moreover, she
slept diagonally on the bias, from the right corner at the
head of the bed to the left corner at the foot. Unless she was
able to "control" the bed-space in this way, she felt insecure.
Unfortunately, this sleep position made it difficult for male
friends to stay overnight with her, since they were invariably
squeezed out of bed.

It struck me that this need to control the bed-space seemed
to be a nighttime carry-over from her waking activities. In
her day-to-day relationships with men she also tried to dominate the situation as much as possible, psychologically squeez-
ing her male friends out of the center of her life. As a result
of this imperialism, her whole existence was skewed—just as
in her sleep period. In effect, she lived on the bias. The correlation between her sleep position and her general way of
living was so striking that I became curious whether similar

9

correlations might exist for other of my patients. And, indeed, this proved to be the case.

During my interviews with patients, I began to elicit and take note of not only the usual material concerning their history, symptoms, relationships, fantasies and dreams, but also this new category of data—their sleep positions. In psychotherapy sessions, it is common for some patients to have difficulty relating to the intellectual rigors of such techniques as dream interpretation, but I found that almost all patients had strong, direct reactions to the concept of sleep positions. Their interest and enthusiasm brought such productive results that I was encouraged to investigate further, and to make more and more use of the information gathered on the subject.

Most patients, I discovered, had considerable awareness of their sleep position. Those who were not immediately certain about how they slept were quickly able to determine their positions once their attention had been drawn to the idea. It is obviously a simple matter to take note of the position assumed on first getting into bed at night. But it is also easy to determine the positions taken at other times during the sleep period. We may wake briefly at various times in the course of the night, and by becoming aware of how we are lying when we wake at these moments, we can soon discover the unique bodily configurations each of us adopts while asleep. Similarly, we can take note of the position in which we find ourselves upon first waking in the morning.

The accuracy with which an individual can determine his or her generally preferred sleep position—even down to such details as whether the ankles are crossed and how the hands are placed—is very high. In many cases, I was able to corroborate the information given me by patients through the objective reports of spouses or friends who shared a bed or bedroom with the patient. Readers of this book can use the same method to check the accuracy of their own awareness. It might also be instructive for the reader to make some guesses about the meanings of various sleep positions.

As my own interest in sleep positions grew, I looked into the psychoanalytic and behavioral literature on the subject, and discovered that very little pertinent material existed. Alfred Adler did attach a brief note concerning sleep posture to a 1914 paper on the problem of insomnia. The note stated in part: "A careful examination based on extensive data will certainly show that the *sleeping posture* of a person indicates his guiding-line." He respectfully invited "psychiatrists, neurologists and teachers to increase this list of sleeping postures," adding that an understanding of sleep positions might well have "great significance for teaching." As we shall discover, the potential significance extends far beyond Adler's limited assumption.

One of Adler's students, Suzanne Schalit, responded to his invitation, and in 1925 published a paper on sleep positions in children and adults, focusing particularly on case studies of children. This paper was based on the rather special psychoanalytic theories of Adler, however, so that its usefulness is somewhat restricted. In the sparse literature on the topic, I also found an interesting 1931 paper by a Heidelberg neurologist, H. Thorner, dealing with the relationship between sleep positions and various neurological responses. The chief American work on the subject was done in the 1930's at the Mellon Institute in Pittsburgh—a project undertaken for the Simmons Mattress Company by H. M. Johnson. The Mellon study and some later studies derived from it were, however, concerned only with the physiology of sleep movements and positions, rather than with their behavioral significance.

In fact, a comprehensive analysis of sleep positions, their meanings, and their relationship to other phenomena of sleep has not previously been attempted. Despite the publication over the past two decades of more than six hundred papers a year by sleep researchers, there has been virtually no discussion of sleep positions. Most studies have involved the recording of technical data concerning the activities of the brain and body during sleep. An understanding of the major discoveries resulting from these studies is vital.

But it is only by combining this information with the special significance of sleep positions that we can finally arrive at a complete picture of the "sleep world"—a world which, when fully understood, extends our perception of the range of human experience and adds new perspectives to our awareness of ourselves as human beings. The practical applications of this new concept of the sleep world are manifold, providing us with fresh approaches in many areas, from couple relationships to the problem of insomnia. What our sleep positions tell about us is not merely revealing—it can help us to deal more cogently with the whole of our existence, both waking and sleeping.

For his editorial assistance in the preparation of this book on the phenomenon of sleep positions, I am grateful to John Malone.

I also wish to express my thanks to Lee Mackler, librarian of The Postgraduate Center for Mental Health, for her help in the survey of the literature.

CHAPTER

I

THROUGH THE
TWILIGHT ZONE

I CALLED HIM the Envelope Man.

A former patient of mine, the Envelope Man had an extremely complex ritual that had to be carried out to the last detail each night in order for him to get to sleep. Before he got into bed, he would arrange on his night table the following items: an opened bottle of Coca-Cola with a glass ready for action, a pack of cigarettes, a lighter and a nasal spray. The covers on the bed had to be tucked in so there wasn't the least crease showing, and the sheet had to be pulled up as tightly as possible, like a veritable swaddling cloth. Into this envelope of bedclothes he would insert himself as neatly as a piece of notepaper. Even when traveling, he found it necessary to carry the entire array of bedside paraphernalia with him and to arrange the bed coverings in the same precise way. In the course of a night, he would usually awaken, fill the glass with Coke and drink, light a cigarette, smoke, and finally use the nasal spray. This ceremony accomplished, he would then feel secure enough to sleep through the remainder of the night.

The behavior of the Envelope Man was extreme, but all of us to one degree or another go through nightly rituals to prepare ourselves for entry into the sleep world. Even our most ordinary, straightforward pre-sleep activities—undressing, brushing our teeth, urinating, putting on pajamas or a nightgown, turning off the lights—are carried out by each of us according to a general pattern that is unique to the individual. A husband may brush his teeth before undressing, his wife after putting on her nightgown. Bedroom lights will be turned off in a particular order, night after night. And if a certain critical aspect of the ritual is neglected, most people will get up again out of bed to remedy the oversight, opening the window or filling the water glass or placing a packet of tissues within reach. The individual who decides that he is too tired to get up and complete the overall ritual will often, in spite of his fatigue, find himself unable to sleep until he finally complies with the need to have everything in its proper place.

Although there is sometimes an eccentric aspect to our pre-sleep rituals, they are important for several reasons. For one thing, their habitual, automatic nature assists us in withdrawing ourselves and our thoughts from the activities of the day world. The motions we go through are so much a part of us that we could "do them in our sleep." Since we don't have to think about what we are doing, these actions are deeply soothing, helping us to achieve physical and emotional tranquillity.

But there is more to it than that. The Envelope Man was not merely calming himself. He, like all of us, was reassuring himself that the day world, the ordinary waking world of work, of social and other relationships in which he took part, would be there during sleep and that he would find it still there when he awoke in the morning—or even in the middle of the night. The need to feel sure of the continuing existence of these relationships shows itself particularly in people suffering from depression and related disturbances. Such people often have difficulty sleeping; they are afraid of losing touch with the waking world, of being separated from the landscapes of their familiar "lived" environments, and thus fear sleep itself. Often it is not until dawn, when the rising sun gives explicit visual evidence that the world is still there, that some individuals can feel sufficiently secure to allow themselves to sleep soundly. While such anxieties concerning sleep are an indication of problematic life situations, none of us is completely free of the awareness that when we pass into the sleep world we are relinquishing one kind of life, a reassuringly known routine, and venturing forth into a completely different state of being.

Sometimes we require specific objects to reassure ourselves. In Czarist Russia, the nobility usually went to bed with a small pillow called a *doumka*—which means "the one you tell your thoughts to." Like the security blanket constantly dragged around by Linus in the "Peanuts" cartoon strip, such objects can take on an exaggerated psychological importance. Why should we need such seemingly silly, childish things to help us sleep? Everyone knows that sleep is not only beneficial but necessary. Sleep deprivation experiments, in which subjects are prevented from sleeping for long periods of time, have shown that to deprive a person of sleep over a number of days has far more serious consequences than to deprive him of food, causing a progressive loss of ability to solve even simple mental problems and leading eventually to increasing signs of delirium. Since we spend so much time sleeping, and fully recognize its importance to the healthy functioning of our waking selves, it may seem paradoxical that sleep should be in any way threatening, or that we should need special objects or comforting ceremonies to help us prepare for it.

Yet sleep has always held complex meanings for mankind.

On the one hand, it is the repose that restores us, a nightly rebirth, giving us the renewed strength to deal with the stresses and to enjoy the pleasures of our waking existence. At the other extreme, *The Big Sleep*, as in the Humphrey Bogart film of that name, is death. In many cultures, in fact, the process of drifting off to sleep is understood in terms of a myth in which the soul temporarily passes out of the body. In some societies it is believed that during sleep the soul wanders in a disembodied state through a kind of limbo; in others it is thought that the soul takes on an alternate form, either animal or human. Many tribal cultures have specific taboos about disturbing the sleeping mat of a person who is away on a hunt or at war, fearing that the spirit will not have a place to return to and that the hunter will therefore die.

Sleep, then, is far more than a mere physical necessity. It is an unknown cosmos—with its own special dimensions of space, time and sensation—that we enter into once every twenty-four hours. As we prepare for bed, each of us becomes a Columbus of the dark, setting out to "the ends of the night." It is only reasonable that we should therefore feel a need to reassure ourselves before embarking on our nightly voyage of discovery, to prepare ourselves psychologically for leaving the day world behind.

The basic rhythm of the human day, called the circadian rhythm, reflects the planetary movement of the earth itself, turning upon its axis as it revolves about the sun. "Circadian" derives from the Latin words *circa dies,* literally meaning "around the day." Like his closest relatives, the apes, monkeys and chimpanzees, the human is a diurnal animal, a creature of daylight, as distinguished from such nocturnal beings as cats, owls and moths. Humans can adjust to sleeping by day and working by night, but our natural inclination is to be active during the day and to rest at night. By day we occupy a visual world in which objects have sharp definition, depth, color and texture. In the daylight a man can *see* the difference between a bush and a wild animal, but in the dark they are both vague forms without explicit shape, if they can be seen at all. From humanity's earliest beginnings, therefore, the day was for dealing with a universe of concrete objects, for hunting, for tilling the fields, for making tools, while the night, in which no work was possible, formed a natural pause between the activities of one day and the next, a time for sleep. The sleep world itself is a timeless, spaceless, formless, seemingly endless void. In the course of the night, as we sleep, we periodically populate the void with the myriad people, objects, sights, and sounds that are our dreams. Both worlds—the daylight world of shape and substance, and the formless sleep world—are equally real, different as they may seem.

In every twenty-four-hour period, each of us experiences the two separate realities of these worlds. For most of us, the twenty-four-hour cycle has now been divided into three periods of diminishing activity. Beginning in the morning, there is first a period of work, generally coinciding with maximum daylight, followed in the evening by an interim period during which we begin to put aside the concerns of the day world, and finally there is a period of sleep. As the work day has become steadily shorter with the growth of technology, the interim period between work and sleep has correspondingly lengthened. In modern life, this interim period is commonly given over to one form or another of relaxation and entertainment, allowing the individual gradually to withdraw from involvement with the stimuli of the work world.

As the interim period itself draws to a close, we slow down

our activities, and our attention is now turned more and more toward our self and toward our immediate environment, as we restrict ourselves first to the area of the home and then later the bedroom and finally the bed. Paralleling this narrowing of the scope of our physical environment, the psychological focus of our awareness also changes, shifting away from the multiple concerns of the day world and becoming increasingly centered upon our own bodily being.

We begin to feel tired. This means that the sleep centers of the brain are activated and have begun to send out the chemical and neurological messages calling our being to rest. Now the natural reflex of yawning sets in as we attempt to obtain more oxygen in order to revitalize the body. During the slight struggle that ensues between our inclination to move on into the sleep world and the attempt to stay awake, we may stretch in an effort to stimulate our slackening muscles. Laughter is frequent at this stage of the evening; as with yawning, we take in extra oxygen when we laugh, but at the same time our laughter is relaxing, a phenomenon of release.

At this point we begin to enter what I call the *twilight zone* between waking and sleeping. It is in this twilight zone, as the sleep centers of the brain gradually come to dominate our physical and psychological processes, that the final important events occur preparatory to actual sleep.

We decide that it is time for bed. We go through the rituals of washing and undressing. We may put on special garments, donning a new garb appropriate to sleep. Finally we get into bed, moving from the vertical perspective of the day world to the horizontal position of the night world, changing from an orientation of maximum mobility to one of maximum inactivity. With this change from a vertical to a horizontal perspective, the range of our vision also has new limits placed upon it, encouraging us to shut and seal our eyelids—our biological sleep shades. And now, ready to move on into the night world, we assume the habitual body position in which we find it easiest to surrender to sleep.

In later chapters, I will be discussing in detail the variety and significance of the positions that we assume while falling asleep, as well as those taken during sleep and in the process of waking. But before the meanings of such sleep positions can be fully explored, it is necessary to understand the specific physical and psychological settings and processes that govern the world of sleep, from the time we first enter the twilight zone, on through the various stages of sleep we experience each night, until we wake the next morning.

The environmental setting, the stage upon which the events of our sleep experience are enacted, is the bed. "The bed, my friend, is our whole life," wrote Guy de Maupassant. "It is there that we are born, it is there that we love, it is there that we die." And it is there also, in this place so central to the human experience, that we encounter the separate world of sleep.

For our primitive ancestors, the earliest men, the bed was no more than a small excavation in the ground, surrounded by a pile of dirt or leaves. But even at this early stage of human development, the chosen sleeping place was imbued with many characteristics that remain with us today.

First, it reflected the concept of territoriality; it was an area with a kind of psychological fence around it, that belonged to the person who had chosen it. We don't just think of "the bed" but of "my bed," or, as couples, of "our bed." This territorial aspect of the bed is also common among many animals. Gorillas, for instance, define their sleeping areas through the use of a fence of leafy boughs.

Secondly, even in its most primitive forms, the bed had to be a place of safety, in which it was possible to feel secure. In the absence of such a feeling of security, sleep is difficult. This is also true for animals. Although elephants usually sleep lying down on their sides, a sick elephant will sleep standing up because it would not feel secure in the prone position—in its weakened state, the extra time and effort of getting to its feet in an emergency would make the animal more vulnerable.

Among primitive peoples living out of doors, safety from attack, whether by dangerous predators or human enemies, is a first consideration in choosing a place to sleep. Yet even within the steel and concrete walls of the modern high rise, the bed remains a place of ultimate security. Almost everyone at one time or another has reacted to stress by "taking to bed." There are numerous cases of individuals whose attachment to the bed has reached pathological proportions. Proust, for example, rarely left his bedroom during the many years he spent writing *Remembrance of Things Past*. Oblomov, the eponymic hero of Ivan Goncharov's novel, spent most of his life in bed. For both of these men, one real and the other fictional, staying in bed made it less necessary for them to face the complexities of the day world. And while the vast majority of us look upon our beds primarily as a place for sleeping and not as a permanent retreat from the world, the associations with security are built up in us from the cradle.

If the bed is to be used as a retreat, of course, it must offer considerable comfort. Although it seems unlikely that there were many Prousts or Oblomovs among early human societies, living out their days languishing upon piles of leaves, the search for comfort in our beds is a third characteristic that mankind has been preoccupied with from the very beginning. Gradually, as ancient societies developed, rude sleeping platforms were devised, sometimes constructed of wood, sometimes of interwoven strips of hide stretched on a framework. The hammock also was used very early in history. Sleeping arrangements among primitive peoples were to a large extent communal, with many members of the family or tribe sleeping in the same cave, tent of animal skins or wooden lean-to. This practice not only provided additional safety, but in colder climates allowed for the most effective utilization of human body warmth, a feature still important among the Eskimos.

It is not until recent centuries that we begin to see the development of the modern bedroom as we know it, at least for ordinary people. Until the fifteenth century, a separate room for sleeping was the prerogative of kings; the peasantry usually slept in the same large room where they cooked and ate, often sharing it with their livestock as well. Indeed, as though to emphasize how privileged such separate sleeping accommodations were, royalty frequently conducted much of their public business while lying down, with members of the court or petitioners being ceremoniously ushered into the bedchamber or a council chamber provided with a royal couch. During the fourteenth century, the French king Louis XI even appeared before Parliament lounging upon a bed on a raised dais.

As the bedroom itself became commonplace during the fifteenth and sixteenth centuries, the next step was to provide different sleeping rooms for different members of the family, separating the children from their parents through the night. This development emphasizes the private nature of the sleep world. In the United States, this practice has been carried further than in any other society, and many psychologists feel that this factor has an important bearing on the particularly independent nature of Americans. Many children do not take well to being left alone in a room of their own, however, and require the ritual reading of bedtime stories or the presence of a favorite stuffed toy to lull them into sleep.

For many people, as they enter each night into the twilight zone between waking and sleeping, the physical nature of the bed itself becomes important. All of us usually experience difficulty in adjusting to a different, unknown bed and bedroom. For some, the pillows, the number of blankets, even the kind of cloth of which the sheets are made can take on importance. The all-time pillow champion was the great tenor, Enrico Caruso, who slept surrounded by as many as eighteen of them. Even the placement of the bed in the room is of concern to many people. When Charles Dickens toured America in the 1840's, he always rearranged the furniture in his hotel bedroom so that the head of the bed was pointing due north according to a compass that he carried with him. The great author was in thrall to a theory of the time that magnetic currents running back and forth between the north and south poles should be allowed to follow their natural path through the bed itself if the occupant was to sleep well.

In addition to the question of how the bed is placed, or how many pillows are necessary for comfort and security, temperature is an important element affecting our relaxed entry into the sleep world. An abrupt immersion in chilled sheets is likely to shock the body into wakefulness once again. To combat excessive coldness, people used to place hot bricks wrapped in flannel or hot water bottles in the bed. With central heating and electric blankets, such devices became unnecessary.

Although a cold bed is unpleasant, a certain degree of coolness is conducive to falling asleep. In fact, as we fall asleep the body itself cools, our temperature dropping an average of two degrees in the course of the night. The need to maintain a comfortable body temperature obviously affects what we wear to bed. In cold climates, flannel may be necessary, but in temperate climates we dress ourselves in lightweight clothing. In hot areas of the world people sleep either nude or wearing as little as possible. The men of India, for instance, wear a *charpoy,* a kind of loincloth or narrow wrap around the hips, and the women wear extremely thin saris.

"Do you sleep in the nude?" is a favorite question of journalists and gossip columnists when interviewing movie stars and other celebrities, although the public's interest in the answer has more to do with sexual curiosity than with human comfort. Nude sleeping has in fact been common at various times throughout human history. Seventy percent of American men sleep in the nude, but only 30 percent of the women—although these statistics predate the women's liberation movement. During the Middle Ages, surprisingly, nude sleeping was the approved custom. A fourteenth-century account cites as proof of his eccentricity the fact that a man went to bed wearing his shirt and drawers. The trend to elaborately decorated sleeping garments in the Renaissance and later appears to have been motivated chiefly by a concern with fashion and status rather than sleeping comfort.

While nude sleeping may be the most comfortable mode of passing the night in a well-built house, it can present real problems to people of tropical countries whose rudimentary dwelling places offer only minimal protection against the numerous natural pests of the jungle or grassland. Certain tribes in the Niger area of Africa sleep in pits of charcoal dust, for instance, since the charcoal residue is supposed to keep away the flying and crawling disturbers of sleep.

In other societies, the great scourge of sleep has always

been the bedbug. The biting of these minute creatures can bring even the most tired of men cursing and scratching back from the twilight zone to full wakefulness. In past centuries, the nobility often required a servant to get into bed before they did, acting as a human hors d'oeuvre long enough to satisfy the bedbugs' hunger, so that the noble could slip into bed and fall asleep undisturbed by the temporarily satiated tiny tormentors. One of the secondary benefits of the industrial revolution of the nineteenth century was that mass-produced bedsteads of brass and other metals did not contain the cracks and crannies of wooden beds in which the insects so happily hid themselves away. But as most travelers on a budget have learned to their discomfort, the bedbug may still be found in its native habitat in cheap hotels the world over.

We must have a secure place to sleep.

We must be comfortable—cool but not cold, warm but not hot. Our sleeping garments or lack of them, the kinds and number of coverings on the bed itself, are regulated to control that comfort.

Beyond that we require a certain degree of darkness for sleep. We close the shutters, pull down the shades and turn out the lights. The darkness of the room in which we spend the night is an important aid to falling asleep and staying asleep. In a room without curtains, we will certainly awake earlier in the morning than if the dawn light is shut out. Sleep is possible under glaring light conditions, but laboratory tests have shown that such sleep is neither as profound nor as refreshing. Being diurnal creatures, the presence of light is a stimulation inevitably associated with the day world; in the dark it is far easier to put aside the concerns of the waking world.

Lying in bed with our eyes closed, we take leave of the day world with its rich panorama of people, objects, colors, actions and distant horizons—and enter a world in which we "see" with our thoughts rather than our eyes. Our minds are still active, but in a different way, drifting from one thing to another. We are in the midst of the pre-sleep reverie, a state halfway between the daydream and the true dreams of actual sleep. As the sharp daytime focus of our thoughts diminishes, this period of reverie becomes for some people a time of great creativity. Many famous artists and philosophers have found the twilight period to be an interval in which new ideas or solutions to old problems suddenly spring to mind.

Philosophers themselves have been of two minds about sleep. Immanuel Kant resented having to sleep, considering it a necessary evil and dreaming a waste of time. To him the night world was one in which he wished to linger as short a time as possible. The thrifty American philosopher Benjamin Franklin also resented sleep, and his famous dictum, "Early to bed and early to rise, makes a man healthy, wealthy and wise," reflects his preference for the day world of concerted action. The great seventeenth-century French philosopher Descartes, however, spent a large part of his life in bed, and it was there that he conceived many of the elements of his philosophy. Hobbes, the English philosopher of the same period, did much of his thinking in bed, and is reported to have scribbled his ideas and mathematical formulae on the bedsheets and even on his own thighs.

For most of us, however, the twilight zone acts as a kind of decompression chamber in which the day world is gradually left further and further behind, while the night world becomes more and more completely enveloping. As we pass from the day world to that of the night, we become more and more focused on our own body. In the twilight zone we become aware of our internal organs in a way that is quite different from daytime experience. We have an increased awareness of the two-step beating of the heart, systole and diastole, as it pumps the blood through its chambers. We sense the previously obscured functioning of other internal organs, such as the lungs and the digestive tract. The weight of our musculature seems more pronounced, and the position of our arms and legs becomes the focus of our attention. The muscles of the trunk of the body lose some of their tone, as do those of the larger muscle groups of the arms and legs. Our heads sink deeper into the pillow as the neck muscles supporting the head relax. In the day world our muscles must always be standing at attention, as it were, ready to be called to instant action; but as our entry into the sleep world progresses we can allow them to lie at ease, to rest.

Paralleling this increased sense of our own body, changes are also taking place in the brain. Most of the scientific evidence we have concerning sleep has been developed in the past two decades, following the discovery in 1953 by Aserinsky and Kleitman of rapid eye movement (REM) as characteristic of dreaming sleep. Using this phenomenon as an indicator, Dement and others doing research in sleep laboratories in the United States and throughout the world have uncovered important, fundamental, and sometimes startling data about dreaming, sleep, and related biological and psychological functions. One of the findings of such research was that as we enter more deeply into the twilight zone, the brain waves characteristic of waking activity slow down, taking on a new, more regular relaxed configuration known as *alpha rhythm*. The brain waves show varying patterns throughout the night, and in the next chapter we will be exploring more fully their nature and significance.

As the alpha waves begin to be emitted by the brain, our

blood pressure also falls slightly, the heart beats more slowly, our breathing becomes less rapid and more regular, the workings of the gastrointestinal system proceed at a slower rate, and the activity of many of our glands changes. Our temperature drops. In certain animals the slowing down of the body processes is so great that not just nocturnal sleep but the seasonal sleep of hibernation is possible. Some hibernating fish such as the carp, being cold-blooded, undergo a temperature drop to 1 degree below freezing; they can actually remain alive at this temperature, even though for all practical purposes they are frozen solid.

Because we are warm-blooded creatures and less tightly bound to our environment, the changes in our own vital processes are of course more limited. But, as we have seen, our physical processes do partake of the shift from the day world to the night world. As we reach the end of the twilight zone, hovering at the edge of true sleep, our thoughts also take on a new form.

As our experience of the twilight zone deepens and intensifies, we have quick visual flashes, images that are, however, unlike the dreams of full sleep. If we compare the sleeping dream to an absorbing movie with continuing action, the images we experience in the twilight zone are more like a slide show. And while the sleeping dream is often fantastic, filled with impossible happenings, the images that appear to us just before the onset of sleep are usually related to our everyday activities. It is assumed by many sleep researchers that these rapid flickering images are an attempt to quickly bind together in a logically integrated way our residual awareness of the day world, even as we are turning away from it to the special experiences of the night world, so that we will then be able to move as smoothly as possible into our actual sleep existence.

The images that normally come to us at this time are called *hypnagogic* hallucinations. Hypnagogic comes from the root words *hypno,* meaning sleep, and *agogic,* meaning leading to. Hypnagogic imagery seems to have no connection with the person who is dreaming about or thinking about or perceiving these fragmented events, even when they are a direct reflection of something we have done or seen during the past day. These recalled experiences of our daily life appear to us as though they were occurring at some remove from where we are now, like a personal television news program wrapping up the highlights of our day that we nevertheless view without a deep sense of personal involvement. As these thoughts and images flicker in the focus of our changing consciousness, our full-scale relationship with the day world is gradually dissolved. And then suddenly, like the last light being extinguished at sunset, the day world is gone altogether.

We are no longer a part of that day world; we have come out on the other side of the twilight zone and now exist only in the night world.

We are asleep.

CHAPTER
II

IN THE SLEEP
WORLD

IN THE TWO DECADES since the discovery of the correlation between rapid eye movements (REMs) and dreaming, there have been many other revelations about sleep. Sleep researchers have developed their data with the aid of an instrument called the electroencephalograph, which detects the faint electrical impulses of the brain and records them in the visual form of an electroencephalogram, or EEG for short. Much as a stereo system amplifies the impulses that have been etched into a phonographic record, and then passes this information on to the speakers in the form of recognizable sound, so the electroencephalograph translates our brain waves into graphic patterns that the researcher can see and understand.

Whether we are awake or asleep, the brain constantly sends off a variety of electrical impulses. If we are working, our brains will give off one kind of impulse. In states of relaxation, alpha waves like those of the twilight zone will be produced. If we are asleep, still other patterns appear, varying according to the particular stage of sleep we are in. The pens of the EEG machine record these changing impulses on a moving strip of paper, in the form of scratchy lines or waves. A formal system of sleep stages, based on these wave patterns, has been adopted—it comprises four different stages of non-

32

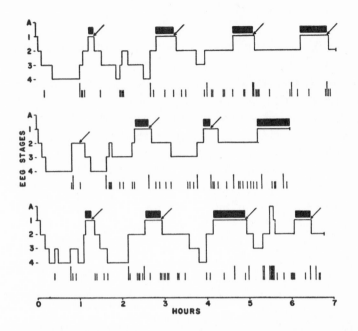

Plots of EEG stages during three nights. The *thick bars* above the EEG lines indicate periods during which rapid eye movements were seen. The *arrows* indicate the end of one EEG cycle and the beginning of the next. The vertical lines below each plot stand for body movements. The longer lines indicate large movement, changes in position of the whole body; the shorter lines represent small movements.

rapid eye movement (NREM) sleep, and a stage of REM dreaming sleep.

In the course of our journey through the night world, we pass in and out of these sleep stages in four to six recurring cycles, depending upon how long we sleep. Each cycle lasts about ninety minutes and is composed of a NREM phase followed by a REM phase. (See graph, Typical Sleep Stages, showing the architectural pattern of the sleep graph.)

Using the EEG and various instruments that measure eye movements, muscle activity, respiration and other functions, sleep research has thus established a clear outline of the sleep experience. On the basis of this knowledge, we can now map out the peaks and valleys of our voyage through the night. We can describe in detail the phenomena we experience during the part of our lives spent in sleep.

What happens to our senses in the sleep world? How much can we hear? What are the motions of our eyes as we "watch" our dreams unfold? When do we move in the night, changing our positions?

We are asleep.

The twilight zone is behind us, and we have entered fully into the sleep world. We could still be awakened easily at this point, and if we were we might insist that we had been awake all along. But something remarkable has happened to us, even though we are unaware of it. We have become functionally blind.

In normal waking activity our eyes move constantly; like the twin muzzles of a shotgun, they swivel together in unison. These coordinated eye movements gradually slow down as we pass through the twilight zone; the pupils narrow, shutting out light. By the time we enter the sleep world, our eyes are moving with slow rolling motions. Experiments have shown that if the eyelids are taped open, and a light flashed in the eyes, the subject will not register or remember it once he is asleep. This exact test of functional blindness has been carried out many times in sleep laboratories. Anyone who has ever had a cat or a dog has seen for himself the evidence of functional blindness in animals. A dog asleep on a couch may have its eyes open, but if a hand is waved in front of its face, the dog will not react. In fact, it is not unusual for human beings also to sleep with their eyes open—it can be observed in soldiers on night sentry duty, for instance.

Once we are asleep, therefore, we are not likely to be disturbed by light. But a sharp, unusual sound might very well waken us again. Noise itself will not necessarily disturb our sleep, or keep us awake, however. We can learn to sleep through the clamor of construction on a new building next door, once we get used to it. Soldiers can sleep on the battlefield in spite of the booming of guns. Some people actually sleep best in the presence of certain kinds of noise, and will prefer to fall asleep with the radio or television on. In a newspaper interview, a young San Francisco woman spoke of being unable to fall asleep unless she was listening to rock music—since the loud music disturbed her parents, she resorted to wearing earphones to bed.

But although we can sleep in noisy conditions, and may even in some cases require them, we are selective about the sounds we respond to when we sleep. Some kinds of familiar noise may not disturb us in the least, may even soothe us, but a sudden unfamiliar noise will waken us immediately. It is almost impossible to creep up on an animal asleep in the wild or even in zoos. Similarly, human hearing also remains alert throughout the night to sounds that are out of the ordinary. The parent who automatically wakens at the cry of a baby in the next room demonstrates the sensitivity of our hearing during sleep.

Sleep often begins with a jerk, like the starting up of a train or bus. This sudden twitching movement that occurs in stage 1 of NREM sleep is called a *myoclonic jerk,* and is caused by an abrupt flare-up of electrical activity in the brain. The myoclonic jerk is like a miniature version of an epileptic attack, but it is an altogether normal part of the sleep world. In most cases, we are unaware of its occurrence, and our body relaxes again as we continue our journey into the night.

We now enter fully into the first two stages of sleep. In stage 1, light sleep, the EEG will show a pattern that looks like a row of *m*'s written in fast cramped scribble. We remain in this stage only about five minutes. Then the brain waves change again with the onset of NREM stage 2. In a sleep laboratory, the pens of the EEG machine would be recording in rapid bursts a new pattern resembling a wire spindle. Stage 2 seems to be a transition between the first stage of light sleep and the more profound sleep to come in stage 3 and stage 4.

The sleep world now utterly encloses us, and we are carried toward the unbounded horizon. Stages 3 and 4 are both characterized by the presence of large, rolling, slow brain waves. If one compares the brain waves of waking activity to the small, rapid, rippling waves at the ocean shoreline on a windy day, the slow waves of stages 3 and 4 could be described as the kind of high unfolding breakers ideal for surfboarding. These slow waves never appear during waking activity in normal people, although they are sometimes found in an individual who has suffered brain damage. Here again, we have a clear indication of how fundamentally different the physiology of sleep is from that of waking.

The waves of stages 3 and 4 are *synchronized*—unlike those of waking activity. When one is awake, the brain must deal with so many different, sometimes sudden and often complex activities at once that the waves recorded on the EEG are *de-synchronized,* appearing in rapid irregular bursts as different parts of the brain go about their separate tasks. But the more fully asleep one is, the fewer functions requiring alertness and concentration there are for the brain to control. As a result, the waves gradually become more and more synchronized in fully relaxed sleep, indicating that both body and brain are smoothly purring away like an idling engine.

We are now profoundly asleep. We have very little eye movement. Our body is thoroughly at rest in a given sleep position. And yet something new is happening, something that doesn't happen while we are awake. The supply of certain biologically active chemicals of the amine family are beginning to increase and to be stored in various cells and cell parts of the brain tissue. If we don't get enough sleep, this buildup will not occur as regularly as it should—which is one reason why depriving us of sleep over long periods of time has a debilitating effect on our functioning.

As we sleep, other physiological processes go into effect. Various hormones begin to be produced, some of which are drawn upon for a number of biological uses during sleep, while others are stored up by the body for future, waking needs. Research concerning the biochemical processes of the body during sleep is the focus of many experiments currently being carried out by sleep scientists. It is a new field, and there is still a great deal that is not known or understood. But we do know, for instance, that the antibodies that fight infection are produced in greater numbers during sleep. When we are at rest, the body is free to concentrate upon these restorative processes, and it is for this reason that getting plenty of sleep is still the best prescription for us when we are ill.

Yet, beyond all these activities of the sleeping body and brain, there is still another aspect to sleep. As we proceed through the full cycle, the stages of NREM sleep alternate at predictable intervals with another fundamentally different kind of sleep—REM or dreaming sleep. Some dream activity may take place during the NREM phase, but such dreams are not of the bizarre, phantasmagoric sort typical of REM sleep.

The content of dreams occurring during NREM sleep tends to be more in the nature of waking thoughts, and to involve common, everyday imagery—it may deal, for instance, with a specific problem of office work or with filling out a shopping list for the supermarket. The first REM dreaming period, occurring about ninety minutes after we first fall asleep, is the shortest, generally lasting from five to ten minutes. As we continue our journey through the night, the duration of each successive REM phase increases. The longest, which may continue for more than half an hour, occurs in the morning just before we wake.

In the moments before the start of the night's initial period of dreaming sleep, a shifting of the sleep position takes place. Although some infrequent movement may happen during NREM sleep—particularly among individuals who are sleeping badly because of illness or anxiety—the majority of the large-scale body movements during the night takes place just before and just after each separate REM dream. It does not take place during the dream itself, for while the dream continues the body undergoes a flaccid paralysis. The loss of muscle tone at this time is so extensive that the body is incapable of gross movements. The exact moment at which a cat enters the REM phase can be observed, for instance, by the change in its head position. The posterior neck muscles lose tone almost completely, and the head will suddenly drop down onto the paws with a motion like an old man nodding in his rocker.

It is a little over an hour and a half since we fell asleep. We are about to begin our first dream of the night. We turn in our beds. If the position in which we first fell asleep was semi-fetal, lying on one side with our knees drawn halfway up, we might at this point shift from lying on the left side, to lying in the same semi-fetal position on the right side.

Just before the REM dream begins, the EEG shows bursts of saw-toothed waves, like a row of the printed letter *m*. Now, dreaming, our eyes beneath our closed lids begin to move once more, shifting back and forth in the same quick synchronized motion that characterizes waking activity. This rapid eye movement is likely to reflect the kind of dream we are having. If we dream that we are entering a room full of people, our eyes will move back and forth from side to side, as they would in the day world, viewing the horizontal scene before us. But if we dream that we are flying, our eyes will move up and down in a vertical motion, as though to take in the ground below and the clouds above.

We actually "see" our dreams and follow the unfolding action with our eyes. The significance of this is pointed up by the fact that people who have been blind from birth do not have visual dreams, and thus are unable to "see" their dreams. The congenitally blind person, uses his other perceptual senses—touch, hearing and smell. The tips of the fingers will move in a fluttery motion, attempting to outline the shapes of the objects in their dreams—whether the roundness of a pearl or the length of a stick. Persons who were sighted at birth, and blinded at some later point in life, do of course continue to have visual dreams.

For all of us, whether we can or cannot see, the wiggling of the fingers and of the toes is one of the few motions of which we are capable while dreaming. The trunk of the body, the neck, the eyelids, and the larger muscles of the arms and legs are all affected by the paralysis mentioned earlier in this chapter. Aside from the fingers and toes, and the eyes, the only other body part that shows motion during

REM sleep is the genitals. Both men and women usually experience tumescence during the REM phase—the penis and the clitoris become engorged and stiffened.

Genital erections during REM sleep have been extensively studied only for the last fifteen years. Previously, it was believed that the erections with which many men awaken in the morning were caused by bladder pressure, but it has now been established that they correlate with the early morning REM period, the longest of the night. We know now that erections occur, in fact, during each of the REM periods throughout the night, although they can be inhibited by the anxiety associated with nightmares.

The instrument used to verify the presence of genital erections during sleep is a water-filled cuff placed around the shaft of the penis and attached to a pressure recording device. In women, genital erections have been studied in cases of congenital clitoral enlargement, thus enabling the cuff to be used. To give scientific validity to these measurements in women, cases of congenital penile enlargement have also been studied to serve as a comparative control statistic.

These studies have practical application in terms of differentiating between physically based and psychologically based impotence in the male. Physical impotence occurs in cases of nerve damage, as in certain advanced stages of diabetes; it can be treated by implantation within the shaft of the penis of a prosthetic device that can be inflated with fluid to create an artificial erection. Erections occur during REM sleep even though a man may be psychologically impotent in a sexual situation, but cannot take place at all, whether sleeping or waking, if there is organic nerve damage. The true nature of the impotence can thus be established through study of the EEG and the penile erection recording. Then the proper treatment—whether counseling, psychotherapy or sex therapy when impotence is caused by emotional conflicts, or implantation of a prosthetic device in cases of nerve damage—can be prescribed.

The fact that erections occur during the dreaming state can lead to some interesting conclusions in other areas. Premature babies spend 80 percent of their sleeping time in a REM-like state of arousal. Studies suggest that the fetus during the last two months in the womb is in a similar state an even greater proportion of the time—offering the interesting presumption that the fetus then might have a fairly constant genital erection.

At birth, the normal infant spends 50 percent of its sleeping time in the REM state. This percentage steadily decreases as the child matures. In middle adulthood, about 25 percent of the night is passed in REM sleep, and 75 percent in NREM. In the late fifties or early sixties, the amount of REM sleep increases somewhat, but diminishes again at later ages. Erections take place throughout the entire sleeping life of an individual, from the womb to the tomb, and have been recorded as late as ninety years of age.

REM sleep is full of seeming contradictions. Our body is paralyzed, and yet we experience genital erections. We are asleep, and yet we move our eyes as though we could see—indeed, we are seeing our dreams unfold. In addition, during REM sleep there is a reversal of the slowing down of our bodily processes that marks NREM sleep. As we dream, our pulse once again increases, our blood pressure and body temperature rise, we begin to breathe faster and irregularly, our gastric juices and adrenalin flow more quickly. All these functions show considerable activation in REM sleep, equaling waking levels—and sometimes rising to a storm-like intensity that would be indicative of extreme anxiety or even panic if we were awake. It is as though the body senses the possibility of danger in the surrounding environment, and is arousing itself sufficiently to scan that environment without actually waking—like a submarine putting up its periscope to avoid surfacing. This "paradoxical" REM sleep alertness is corroborated by the fact that during this stage our brain waves show a marked similarity to the low, fast, irregular patterns of waking existence. Sometimes, of course, this arousal is accompanied by a nightmare, or triggered by a noise in the night, and we do wake. The formation of gastric ulcers, as well as the occurrence of asthmatic attacks, heart attacks and strokes, are particularly likely during this period of arousal in those individuals susceptible to such illnesses.

In the sleep state we are unaware of the changes taking place in our brains and our bodies. We are not conscious of our own existence in the same manner as by day—we sleep "the sleep of the dead." But in dreaming sleep a special quality of consciousness manifests itself. The universe of our dreams may at some moments be quite similar to the one that our waking self inhabits, and at other moments may be utterly, fantastically different. But we do experience it, are aware of it. If we are wakened while dreaming, we can within the first five minutes report the nature and content of our dreams in great detail. And it is in our dreams that we experience most vividly the unique way of living that characterizes the sleep world.

Psychological studies show that in dreams—as in other altered states of consciousness such as hypnotic trances, certain kinds of religious ecstasies, and drug-induced states—we do not experience a sense of fatigue, nor of strenuous overactivity. No matter what we may be doing in our dreams, we do not feel tired. We may be running—but without the sense of muscular strain or shortness of breath that accompanies the act of running in the waking world.

In the dream world there is a detachment from the realities of a physical self imbedded in a given concrete situation. If, in waking life, we are sitting in a chair behind a desk, we will be acutely aware, in a physical sense, of being in that chair, behind that desk. But in our dreams, we can be sitting in the chair and yet also, at the same time, have the experience of being an onlooker, observing ourselves. There is a sense of our self as being everywhere in the experienced situation. In dreams, the concentration of our attention upon a specific activity is lessened—our perceptual focus is less defined and becomes more encompassing, more cosmic.

Once again we come upon a paradox of the sleep world. While dreaming, we do not make calculated, logical choices based upon the evidence around us, as we generally do in the day world. But this very difference gives us the opportunity for a special freedom of thought. We are free to fly, to become an object, to accomplish impossible tasks. We are free from the constraints of the actual physical world, free from the inhibitions of daily social intercourse. We are free to be completely our own self, to indulge our most private hopes and to face our most secret fears without the camouflages of our daily routine. The dream world is not a distorted derivative of unacceptable day world thoughts. Rather, it is a concrete reality, one in which we can perceive ourselves and the events we create for ourselves in a way that is not usual in the waking world.

In the dream world our perception of space and time becomes quite different. Because we are less able to concentrate our attention on any given fact of our dream environment, we find ourselves in the situation of being responsive to an entire world in which things shade off at the boundaries of our visual experience. It is as though we were living in a cosmos like Einstein's theoretical universe: finite but also unbounded. A man in a sleep laboratory, wakened from a dream, may state that he has climbed twenty steps. Yet under closer questioning, being asked how many steps he actually took, he will answer, "Three." The three steps he has taken in his dream can be physically corroborated by the parallel recording of three upward movements of his eyes, which will have been registered by the instrument keeping track of his eye movements. But the three steps that he took in his dream have brought him, all at once, through a telescoping of action and time, to the top of the flight of twenty stairs.

While dreaming, we are only partially aware of time relationships, so that there is a blending of past, present and future. Our acute waking sense of time structure, as measured by the clock, is diminished. In the dream world, as in waking, we are usually concerned with oncoming events— we are in a given situation from which we look toward an immediate future. But that future can also coexist with a past and a present, all three dimensions of time having become *now*. For instance, we may exist in a dream as a younger self, even a child, but be surrounded by our contemporary, up-to-date environment. When, toward morning, the amount of REM sleep increases, and our dreams become more complex and bizarre, thoughts and images from the past frequently occur as part of our experience of the dreaming present, the *now* of the sleep world.

In dream space, we can exist in a variety of forms. We may in our dreams find that we are a mop, a building, an animal, an anonymous human being, or even ourselves. We can be located in our current home one moment, and a moment later on a South Sea island that we visited ten years ago. Or the two may be brought together, so that we are in a South Sea hut on our own street. We can be in Africa one instant, and on the moon immediately thereafter—even though we have never, in waking life, been either place except in imagination.

The influence of personality shows itself in sleep, not merely in the individual content of dreams, but also in the kind and quality of sleep we get. Creative people and problem solvers—as well as those with neurotic conflicts—generally tend to sleep longer, to have more REM sleep, and to wake up feeling less refreshed than those persons who are down-to-earth. Pragmatic people, who tend to avoid the unclear, the conflictual and the problematic in their waking lives, also do so in the sleep world. Thus they dream less, and experience the paradoxical freedom of image and action in the sleep world less profoundly. On the other hand, they go to sleep rapidly and have less need for long sleep. Since excessive sleep can be as debilitating as too little, such persons may be quite healthy emotionally.

We should not denigrate poor sleepers, however. Many people attempt to solve problems in their sleep, and it is common to hear the phrase, "I'll sleep on that." Many of the greatest discoveries of mankind have been made during sleep or sleep-like states of contemplation and reverie rather than during periods of cold, logical, rationalistic thinking or in controlled experimental situations. Descartes, generally regarded as the father of modern scientific thought, conceived the basic concepts of his work in methodology, mathematics and physics during three separate dreams on one night in 1619.

In the Central Mountain Range of the Malay Peninsula there is a primitive tribe called the Temiar whose members have trained themselves to an astonishing degree to work out their life problems during sleep. Dreams of the previous night are avidly discussed among these people. Under the tutelage of tribal leaders who act as a kind of primitive psychotherapist, tribal members are trained from childhood to attain control over their dream thinking, and even to induce dreams. Through the use of premeditated, programmed dreaming they are able to rid themselves of many kinds of fears and phobias—and as a result, social conflict among these people is virtually eliminated. They are also able to dream of defeating their enemies. The sense of security achieved through the dream victory helps to make actual battle unnecessary. Neighboring tribes are intimidated by the seemingly "magical" powers of this self-confident, dream-based society. Thus, through a kind of psychological warfare, strife with other tribes is forestalled.

Although the Temiar people must be termed "primitive" in a strict anthropological sense, their ability to use their dreams constructively seems a sophisticated talent that many of us in the "civilized" world might well envy, for they make something truly creative of the third of their lives that they spend in the sleep world. They demonstrate that the universe of sleep need not be mere oblivion, that there is more to it than the need for physical rest. In the sleep world we have an opportunity to experience a separate and different world—and it is possible to bring back from that world a knowledge of ourselves that can be of benefit to us in the day world as well.

The most profound sleep, when the usually active brain and body are most deeply involved in restorative functions, is that of NREM stage 4. Stage 4 sleep is concentrated in the first half of the night. In fact, we spend as much time in stage 4 during the first hour and a half of sleep as during the entire remainder of the night. Laboratory experiments thus bear out the old wives' tale that the best sleep of the night is the first. The fact that stage 4 NREM is generally considered the most refreshing sleep we get, and that we get so much of it in the first hours of the night, very likely accounts for the boasts of many famous men that they need only three or four hours of sleep a night. Napoleon, Edison and others may indeed have been able to dispense with the later, less refreshing hours of sleep without an undue sense of fatigue. It is likely, however, that they catnapped at various times during the day.

Experiments have shown that NREM sleep is vital to our healthy functioning in the waking world. A person may be deprived of REM sleep, by waking him each time the EEG indicates that he has begun to dream, without seeming harm. But to prevent the same individual from getting NREM sleep eventually brings on the irritability and loss of mental alertness characteristic of total sleep deprivation.

There is a direct parallel between body size and REM sleep. Birds, for instance, spend only 1 to 5 percent of their sleeping time in the REM phase. The longest periods of REM sleep recorded have been for human beings, elephants and, appropriately enough, the giant sloth. There is considerable evidence to suggest that REM sleep is also related to the scale of evolutionary development. The oldest of earth's land creatures, snakes and other reptiles, have only NREM sleep. Birds, next on the evolutionary ladder, begin to show a small amount of REM sleep. Mammals, which are in relative terms fairly new arrivals on the evolutionary scene, have considerable REM sleep.

The only mammals that do not have REM sleep are two creatures found in Australia and nearby islands, the platypus and the echidna, or spiny anteater. Survivors of a prehistoric class of animals midway on the evolutionary scale between reptiles and mammals, they were apparently saved from extinction by the separation of Australia from the great supercontinent that originally comprised Africa, India and Australia. In an environment free from predators, they have survived to this day. Like mammals, they suckle their young, but like the more primitive reptiles they lay eggs, and their brain patterns remain reptilian, without REM sleep.

Do animals whose brain waves indicate the existence of the REM state actually dream, though?

In a sense there can be only a speculative answer to this question, since the existence of dreams can ultimately be verified solely by a subjective report on the content of a particular dream. But although animals cannot tell us their dreams, the brain waves of horses, elephants, dogs and other animals that have been studied clearly indicate that these creatures spend varying amounts of time in a state that is estimated to be remarkably similar to the REM phase in man. And anyone who has ever wakened a twitching, moaning dog from a "nightmare" has seen for himself the behavioral evidence that animals do indeed have dreams. Horses, which also give signs of having nightmares, sleep standing up in the NREM state, but lie down during REM sleep because of the paralysis that sets in during that phase.

In spite of all the studies that have been made in the last few years concerning the nature of sleep in humans and animals, it is still not known exactly why we need sleep. Pavlov thought that sleep represented an inhibition of the waking brain. Another theory holds that sleep is a kind of switching-off, allowing for a restoration of the bodily processes and chemicals necessary for daytime activity. There is also an intoxication theory of sleep, suggesting that it is caused by the accumulation of some as yet unidentified toxic substance in the body.

Still another approach, the clearance theory, is based on the belief that during sleep a kind of mental chimney sweeping takes place, with unnecessary ideas and memories being eliminated. There is also a reorganizing concept that envisions sleep as a process of repatterning of our thought—this is supposed to take place especially during REM sleep. Finally, there is the conservationist concept, in which sleep is seen as conserving neural energy. In line with this idea, the sentinel function theory suggests that there is a periodic arousal to the threshold of waking during the REM period, allowing the animal (or human) to test the safety of the environment even as sleep continues. No one, however, has yet definitively proven the exact function of sleep. What we do know at present is that sleep is necessary, that there are predictable cyclic activities of the brain and body processes during sleep, and that prolonged lack of sleep has deleterious effects on the behavior of the individual.

The night passes.

We move back and forth through the four stages of NREM sleep, and enter periodically into the REM phase, dreaming our solitary dreams.

As we have seen, there is practically no stage 4 NREM sleep during the early morning hours. Rather we spend most of this period either in REM or in stage 2. The last and longest REM phase of the night begins to usher us back into the day world. Since REM sleep is the closest to actual waking, the long morning period of dreams brings us continually closer to waking consciousness. The body begins to rev up again, with the blood pressure and temperature rising. Our pulse quickens; we breathe more deeply. The wake centers of our brain lose their dampening inhibitions, and begin to arouse us. We again become sensitive to light, and functional blindness ends. The sunlight streaming through the curtains may disturb us, causing us to turn away from it as the final REM period ends and we can move the trunk of our body freely once more. At this point we can make a conscious note of the body position in which we awaken from full sleep. We come half-awake, aware of the morning light, aware, perhaps, of a genital engorgement left over from the final REM period.

We now experience once again the kind of hallucinations that brought us to the threshold of sleep seven or eight hours before. These morning images, however, are of greater duration than those of the twilight zone. We pass in and out of a light, drowsy sleep. "Did you ever see a dream walking?" asks the old song. And yes, all of us have in one sense, for the visual hallucinations of the morning often continue for some moments after we open our eyes.

Only one out of six people is capable of waking spontaneously at a given hour. All of us, of course, are governed by a variety of biological clocks, which we can in some cases preset with will and practice. We become acutely aware of such clocks when we are suffering from jet lag after an overnight trip, or when first working on a night or swing work shift. Few of us are able to tune in our biological clocks with sufficient accuracy to awaken at an appointed hour without the help of a jangling alarm or a tug at the shoulder by a parent, friend, or mate. And many people are able to resist the most persistent efforts to wake them. Adolescents in particular possess a remarkable ability to retreat back into the sleep world, to put off facing the day with its increasingly adult demands.

Oh, how we hate to get up in the morning! At least some of us.

Samuel Johnson, the great eighteenth-century English man of letters, loathed having to get out of bed. With his customary ironic wit, he wrote of his habit of sleeping late: "I have, all my life long, been lying till noon; yet I tell all young men, and tell them with great sincerity, that nobody who does not rise early will ever do any good." Johnson, who liked eating and drinking as much as he did sleeping, was a classic night owl. So far as he was concerned, mornings ought simply to be abolished. But many others, the larks among us, find morning the best part of the day, virtually leaping out of bed, full of instant vitality. But most of us fall somewhere in between these two behavioral extremes. We may not always be thrilled to get up, but we are not "hibernating" bears, either.

As we begin to live in the day world again, mental alertness precedes bodily alertness for most of us. Experiments have shown that when awakened from REM sleep, the majority of people have a surprising degree of mental alertness In many people there is an unusual ability to make word associations, and to think quite creatively at this time. On the other hand, the same subjects, coming out of the limp paralysis of the final REM phase, naturally have difficulty in performing tasks that demand manual dexterity.

Our mental processes have been creatively involved in dreaming, and are already revved up. Our laggard body, however, needs time to shake off the REM paralysis—we must in a sense hoist it up from the horizontal sleep world into the day world, bringing it back into line with the erect vertical orientation of waking existence. For this reason, it is best to take one's first encounter with the vertical world slowly: if you are right-handed, put your right foot out of bed (or your left foot if you are left-handed), and follow it *very slowly* with the other foot. Now you are ready to stand up, and begin again.

CHAPTER

III

BODY IN
THE DARK

A NUMBER OF MY PATIENTS have suffered from a disorder called sleep paralysis. Typically, the patient will awake in the morning and be unable to move. Such patients are back in the day world mentally—they are awake, they know where they are—yet their bodies are still living in the sleep world. The body, in these cases, continues to behave as though it were in the REM phase of sleep. Needless to say, this condition is extremely anxiety-provoking for the patients who suffer from it. There is a discordance between the mental way of living in the day world and the bodily way of being in the night world, with the individual partaking of both worlds at the same time.

Normally, each of us experiences the day world in a whole sense—both our bodies and our thought processes are involved in day-oriented activities. Equally, during our sojourn in the night world, we experience it in a whole way—our mental and body attitudes are both in concert with the sleep state. What the morning sleep paralysis demonstrates is the extent to which the body in the dark is bound to the space on which it rests: the bed. The sleep-paralyzed patient, lying on the bed, is made heavily aware of the body at rest, far more so than we are aware of our bodies when we are standing or sitting erect. When we are erect, the weight of our bodies is absorbed by the springy curvature of the vertebral column and by the cartilaginous cushions of the various joints. Thus to a large extent we are buffered from the evidence of our gravity-bound existence. In sleep, however, we no longer have these natural shock and weight absorbers; as we lie horizontally, every inch of our body experiences at the same time the total pull of gravity upon it. In addition, the proud omnipotence of the head, and of thinking, becomes reduced, so that there is much more equality in the sleep world between the body and the thinking processes.

While the victim of sleep paralysis finds himself mentally in the day world, but bodily still in the night world, this discrepancy between the day and sleep worlds can also occur in the reverse manner. Sleepwalking and sleep-sitting are both examples of the body in the dark behaving as though it existed in the day world, while the individual mentally remains in the sleep world.

During World War II, I myself witnessed an interesting example of sleep-sitting. I was just about to fall asleep, lying in a field hut adjacent to two fellow soldiers. Suddenly, one of them sat up in his sleep, muttering something about "Collins Avenue." Then he immediately fell back again into a horizontal sleep position. At this point, the other soldier also sat up in his bed in his sleep and replied to the first soldier's statement: "Did you say Collins Avenue?" He also lay back down immediately. The next morning, neither of the two soldiers remembered anything about their astonishing sleep conversation.

When individuals suffering from cardiac or respiratory problems find it necessary to sleep sitting up, they usually have difficulty learning to sleep in this upright position—the natural axis of the body in the dark is a horizontal one. In the case of the two soldiers, this horizontal axis was violated by two people within seconds of one another, and an embryonic attempt at day communication also occurred. It can be surmised that the first soldier was sleep-thinking about the Miami Beach training station from which we had just been transferred. In the Miami sun we had had considerable free time, and it had been a much more pleasant situation than the raw field camp where we were now stationed. Remembering Miami and its major thoroughfare, Collins Avenue, in his sleep, the stimulus was apparently strong enough to make the first soldier sit up in bed, attempting to return in a bodily way to that pleasant and familiar day-world scene. His words obviously triggered a similar response in the second soldier.

Sleep-sitting and sleepwalking are often associated with the desire to return to a locale or situation in which the individual previously felt secure, but which is denied him in present circumstances. Another demonstration of this phenomenon concerns a number of my male patients who were children during World War II. They reported to me that they had sleepwalking experiences shortly after the end of the war. While their fathers were away fighting, these young boys were kept in the mother's bedroom during the night, sometimes even sleeping in the same bed with the mother. But once the father returned from the battlefields, the child was banished from the parental bedroom. Trying to return to the longed-for world of their mothers' rooms, these "young lovers"—nicely illustrating the concept of Oedipal rivalry with the father—would walk in their sleep, turning up in the parents' bedroom in the middle of the night.

Sleepwalking does not occur while we dream, of course—that would be impossible because of the paralysis that accompanies the REM state. Rather, it usually occurs during the profound sleep of stage 4. This fact alone clearly indicates that the body in the dark is no mere neutral object at rest, but rather is fully capable of expressing in its way the important relationships of the individual's life. If the person's need to express himself is strong enough, he can behave as though his body were in the day world even during the most inert stage of sleep.

It is best not to wake a sleepwalking person, but simply to lead him gently back to bed. To wake him would make him forcibly aware of the discordance between his mental processes and his bodily activities. Such sudden awareness can be deeply disturbing and anxiety-provoking to the sleepwalker. If he is not awakened, he will not remember the events of his brief excursion in the night. Even as he wanders from room to room the sleepwalker believes himself to be existing in the sleep world—and indeed he is, despite the fact that his body is behaving as though it were in the day world.

There are also individuals upon whom the sleep-world experience lies so heavily that they have difficulty dealing with the day world. As a young doctor, doing my psychiatric residency in a hospital, I became interested in the case of a male patient in his thirties. The man reported that he experienced the illusion that everyone and everything in the world looked tall and thin. He had never learned to give up his babyhood, to stand on his own two feet and cope with the requirements of the adult world. Although he had matured physically, in his thinking and in his life position he had remained essentially an infant. The baby lying in its crib, leading an entirely horizontal life, naturally tends to see everything as extended and tall. This patient, who had never truly moved out of the horizontal life position of infancy, continued to view the world as though looking up from his crib. He was in fact a living example of Oblo-movism, and spent most of his time lying down, expressing with his body the undeveloped way in which he lived.

This is not to say that regularly to assume the horizontal position in the day world is necessarily a mark of personality disturbance. The Medieval and Renaissance kings who received their court while lying on a bed were making a positive rather than a negative psychological statement in taking that position—they were saying to the rest of the world that a king, by the privilege of his rank, might loll at his ease while everyone else must beat a path to his throne. Both the king and the young man in the hospital, however, show that body position is an expression of role and character. The body tells something about an individual; its postures and attitudes are a significant indicator of the person's basic orientation to the world.

In waking life, as we go about our daily tasks, we are fully aware of the meaning of many of the bodily postures and expressions that we encounter in the people around us. Eye contact, gestures, facial mimicry, posture, the positioning of the arms and legs, body attitudes and movement patterns—all offer clues to personality, role relationships, and the emotions of the moment.

Our body expresses our key relationships to people and events. If we change our relationships, then the body will demonstrate in its own way this same change. If we are in an anxious mood, so that the world and the things in it seem threatening, we try to escape the threat by shrinking away. Our body cringes, our extremities are pulled back in fear, our throat tightens. In joy, however, we tend to embrace the world and all its objects. We elevate ourselves in order to gather in as much as we can of life. Our eyebrows rise, our heart throbs more quickly, our breathing is deeper and the chest expands, our mouth lifts at the corners. In sadness, upon hearing of the death of a friend, for instance, we stop moving upward and forward, and just as our thoughts dwell upon the past and our memories of the friend, so everything about our body seems to sag, as though paralleling the dropping of tears from the eyes.

In recent years, as our understanding of how the body expresses relationships, feelings and attitudes in nonverbal ways has grown, body language studies have assumed great importance in the behavioral fields. For instance, one aspect of the behavioral "profile" used to identify potential airplane hijackers at airports around the country, is based on *kinesics* or body language. In another application of kinesics, elementary-school teachers in many areas are provided with information to help them spot the hyperactive child by his unusual body behavior. It is then possible to give these problem children the special attention they need.

It is necessary for therapists involved in group or family therapy to be sensitive not merely to the verbal interchanges among members of the group, but to read the subtle messages conveyed by body attitudes, breathing rates, and other physical evidence. These clues to the understanding of patients are particularly important in the complex interactions of group sessions, with several people often talking at once. In some cases, such group sessions are recorded on film or videotape, so that the interplay among the various members can be more clearly observed.

These techniques for studying human body behavior are centered upon the body as it exists in the day world. Until now, the body in the dark, its special behavior in the sleep world, has been hidden from our attention, and the positions people assume during sleep unnoticed. Studies in sleep laboratories have told us a great deal about what happens in terms of physiological processes during the night. We have learned much over the past two decades about the changes that take place in body functions during sleep, about the significance of genital erections during the REM phase, and we can predict when the body is most likely to move in the course of the night. But these are partitioned observations—they tell us little about the individual's unique personal ways of encountering the sleep world. These studies have treated the body essentially as a chemical or physical organism, and in so doing have overlooked an important dimension of our sleep world experience. In this book, it is my purpose to move beyond the circumscribed technical data about the body in the dark that have already been established, and to show that the particular positions a given person assumes in the course of the night reflect the whole living design of that individual's special life-space, and the way in which he inhabits it.

In order to comprehend the significance of the positions assumed by the body in the dark, it must first be understood that those positions are an extension of the "defensive" behavioral maneuvers that the individual uses in waking life. The concept of defense patterns was one of Freud's important insights. He and later analysts isolated about a score of these *standard discrete* defenses, of which some of the best known are repression, projection and sublimation. If, for example, a person makes use of the tactic of denial as a defense, he will refuse to recognize the meaning of his behavior in a situation even when it is pointed out to him. An analyst might suggest that a patient who is always late to his therapy sessions, but is otherwise prompt, is using this means of expressing his anxiety feelings concerning therapy. The patient, using the denial mechanism, will completely shut his eyes to this interpretation.

There is also a special category of defenses that is comprised of an individual's built-up, habitual, automatic ways of behaving. This type of defense is called a *characterological* one. For instance, a person may typically behave in a passive way. Unassertive and compliant in most of life's situations, he will take on a placatingly submissive posture toward others. A paranoid person will see the world as continually threatening, his eyes always on the alert for signs of potential danger or affront. An aggressive person always has a chip on his shoulder; he leans forward pugnaciously, seeking to overwhelm people and events. These are ways of behaving that the individual feels to be good and necessary, and which he uses without examination.

Both the standard discrete defenses and the characterological defenses are reflected in sleep positions. The standard defenses can be seen in the position one chooses in the twilight zone, as one meets the stresses of this period and tries to relax. I call this preliminary sleep position the *alpha* position. Its exact configuration will, of course, be unique to each individual. A person may, for instance, lie flat on his back with his hands crossed behind his head, the head resting in his palms with the elbows extended like a pair of waterwings. This position indicates that one of the person's standard defenses is that of intellectualization. The cradling of the head (and, by extension, the brain) funnels all perception into the organ of thought. Experience is thereby controlled, stress alleviated, and security established. This sense of security allows the individual to relax, and drowsiness soon sets in.

Some people, whose personalities are less complex or more

rigid than others, may go on to spend most of the night in their chosen alpha position. But the data provided by my case material shows that most people will subsequently change to a second position, usually just as full sleep begins. Knowing that they are about to drift off into the new world of sleep, now completely relaxed, they shift from a position reflecting their standard defenses to one that gives them greater security in their extended encounter with sleep itself —assuming a long-term characterological sleep position. This characterological stance—or *omega* position—generally becomes the preferred one throughout the night. Since the omega position embodies the most fundamental aspects of a person's way of living, all further references to "sleep positions" throughout this book can be taken to mean the omega position unless it is specifically stated that the twilight zone alpha position is being discussed. A person may change positions from time to time during the night, but will regularly return to the dominant, preferred position that reflects his characterological defenses. Usually, he will find himself in that position upon waking in the morning.

The body in the dark, then, is not just *a* body—it is *our own* body. And our body is at all times a part of our own particular way of relating to the world. Every aspect of our body, the functioning of each organ, each tissue, relates more or less directly to those meaningful relationships that constitute our special ways of living at any given time. In fact, as we shall see in later chapters, if we change our ways of living, altering our meaningful relationships, our body too partakes of this new mode of living in the world. Just as the downturned mouth and grieving eyes show the pain of loss in the waking person, so the chosen sleep position will reflect it as well.

Having begun to understand that there is another very real

universe in which we spend a third of our lives—a universe with its own special dimensions of experience—we can now hope to discover, by examining how we live in this universe, a new way of looking at ourselves. And we can expect this new perspective to shed further light on our essential natures.

As we study the passage of the individual from day into night, and through the night into a new day, making note of the particular positions assumed by the body in the dark, we may also be able to see in a clearer way, unclouded by the commerce of daily activity, the crucial, central ways in which each particular person expresses his unique patterns of existence. For the way we sleep reveals the way we live.

CHAPTER

IV

COMMON SLEEP
POSITIONS

A PATIENT OF MINE, a young woman, lies on my psycho-analytic couch, demonstrating her sleep position. She has already described the position verbally, but I have asked her to physically assume it. This serves three purposes. First, it gives her a sense of personal involvement in the interpretive process, serving as a kind of psychodrama. Secondly, it gives concrete corroboration of what she has told me. And it allows me to take note of details that she may not have considered important enough to fully report.

The young woman has assumed one of the four common, basic sleep positions: the *Full-Fetal*. She is lying on her side with her body curled up upon itself, her legs flexed at the knees, the knees drawn up as though attempting to touch her chin. Her entire body is rolled into a kind of ball.

In interpreting the meaning of this sleep position, I do not use a metaphorical or symbolic approach. I deliberately avoid the use of a list of standard symbols with given mean-

FULL-FETAL

ings that is employed in traditional dream interpretation—in which a cup, for instance, is assumed to be a vagina in disguise. Instead of interpreting a cup as a vagina, I would say that to immediate perception a cup is characterized by roundness and depth, and has the properties of receiving, encompassing, enclosing, and of containing fluid.

Similarly, when I look at the full-fetal position, I try to let it speak to me as directly as possible, to let the meanings emerge from the configuration itself. In the full-fetal position, I notice that the individual is lying in a folded position that obscures the face and most of the viscera of the body. This folded position may curve around an object such as a pillow, which serves as a kind of core. Usually, the arms and the hands complete the circle, enfolding the knees or being tucked in in such a way as further to cover the center of the body.

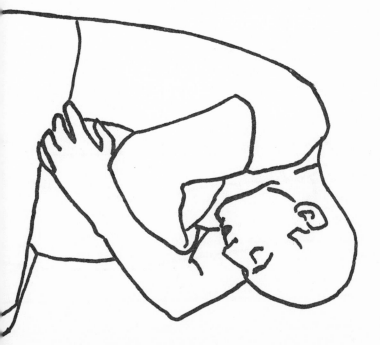

From the essential impression of the sleep position that presents itself to me, I conclude that this individual has not yet allowed herself to unfurl and expose herself to the events of her life. Such a person sleeps and lives like a tightly closed bud, not having allowed herself (or himself) to unfold. The individual resists exposures to the full, open experiencing of life's joys and difficulties.

I also study the position of the sleeper in relationship to the nocturnal domain he or she inhabits, the bed area itself. Individuals who assume the full-fetal position tend to lie mainly in the corners of the bed, usually the upper corners facing outward. In the day world as in the chosen sleep position, such people show a strong desire for protection and the need for a central core around which they can organize their lives and upon which they can depend. They have held themselves rigidly back and cling as closely as possible to a dependent pattern of relationships that afforded them security in the earliest years of their lives.

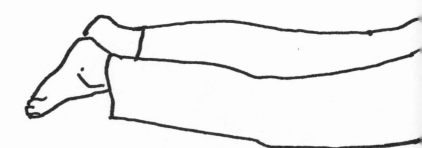

During the several years that I have been studying sleep positions, I have found that the meanings embodied in the given positions strongly correlate with the other known factors about a particular individual. The basic body position a person adopts for reassurance in the sleep world is as indicative of the essential way that person lives as the usual material encountered in therapy sessions: personality characteristics, the attitudes and reactions to myself and important people in their lives, past and present, as well as the material of dreams.

Let us look, for instance, at a second basic sleep position —the *Prone* position. As has already been indicated, the prone position shows an attempt to assume command of the bed-space, to embrace it as fully as possible, making it one's own. By lying facedown on the bed, usually with their arms extended over their heads and their legs stretched out with the feet somewhat apart, prone sleepers show a need to be in touch with—and to regulate—as much of their immediate world as they can. Unless they are able to dominate the bed-space in this way, they feel vulnerable. It is as though by

PRONE

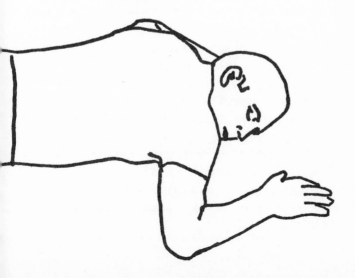

controlling the topography of the bed they will achieve governance over the entire sleep world, protecting themselves from unpleasant surprises in the course of their night's journey.

People who sleep in the prone position show a similar compulsion to regulate the events of their waking lives, the day-to-day environment of their existence. They do not like the unexpected, and organize their lives so as to avoid it whenever possible. For instance, such individuals are almost always on time for appointments, and are disturbed if other people are late. They are fussy about details, neat and exact. If their managerial tendencies are thwarted, they will redouble their efforts to bring the world into line with their own dictates, and thus avoid doubt. Those who feel especially insecure when faced with the unexpected will, like the young woman discussed in the Preface, sleep not only prone but diagonally across the bed, attempting to prevail even more completely over the sleep world.

A third common position is sleeping on the back. An ancient proverb states: "The King sleeps on his back, the Wise Man on his side, and the Rich Man on his stomach." I have found, in fact, that those who sleep in the *Royal* position do generally feel themselves to be the king or queen of their sleep—as well as of their day universe. Such individuals were usually favorite children, or children who always had the center of attention. Many professional theater people sleep in the royal position—perhaps because it is an easy position from which to take a bow and receive the plaudits of the populace. In or out of the theater world, those who sleep in the royal position generally have a security, a self-confidence and a personality strength that makes it possible for them to accept the world and what it has to offer. Awake or asleep, the world is indeed their oyster. They are open to everything, happy to give as well as receive—just as the physical position they assume for sleeping leaves them exposed and open to the night world.

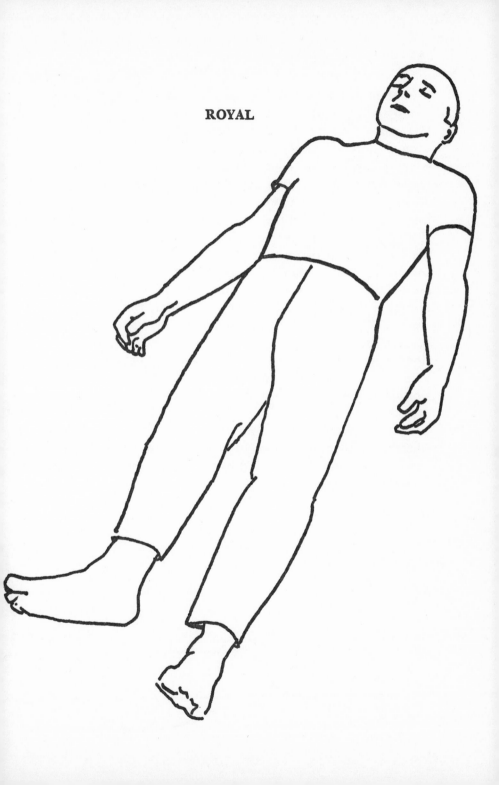

ROYAL

In terms of frequency, the most common position is the *Semi-Fetal*. According to research done by Boris Sidis at Harvard in 1909, 75 percent of those studied who were right-handed slept primarily on the right side—not only while going to sleep but also during the later more profound sleep phases. While the majority did change sides during the night, they showed a distinct preference for the right side if they were right-handed and the left side if they were left-handed.

Sleeping in the semi-fetal position, lying on the side with the knees drawn partway up, has the physical advantage of conserving heat without closing off the circulation of air around the body. Also, the central trunk of the body is protected, especially its psychological center, the heart. The semi-fetal position allows greater maneuverability in the course of the night than any of the other most common positions, since it is possible to turn from one side to the other without undoing the set configuration of the body. The possibilities of movement that still retains the favored position are obviously more limited in the prone or supine positions.

The semi-fetal position thus makes good "common sense" in terms of physical comfort and functioning. The personalities of those who choose this position show a parallel degree of sensible adjustment to the world. Such individuals are

SEMI-FETAL

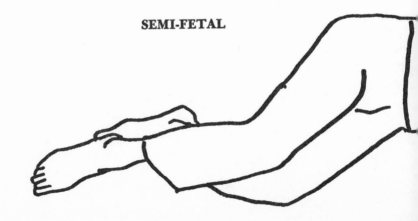

usually fairly well-balanced and secure. They are able to accommodate themselves to the facts of their existence without undue strain. They are not so vulnerable as to feel the need to control the bed-space, nor do they curl tightly around themselves, seeking protection against an uncertain future.

The meaning of these four most common sleep positions is amplified—and often significantly modified—by the positioning of the hands and feet, as we shall see in the next chapter. There are also many variations on the basic positions that will be subsequently explored—for example, the *Sphinx* and the *Swastika* positions, which evolve from the prone position; the *Monkey* and the *Leaner,* which are related to the royal position; as well as the *Mummy* and the *Chain-Gang* variations on the semi-fetal position. It should be further understood that a given person may assume more than one of the basic positions—or related ones—in the course of the night. The average person, when sleeping well, moves twenty to thirty-five times a night. These are gross movements, involving considerable adjustment of the body weight. A person who is ill or sleeping badly because he is extremely anxious or agitated may make more than a hundred major movements a night. And, of course, each of us makes a great many

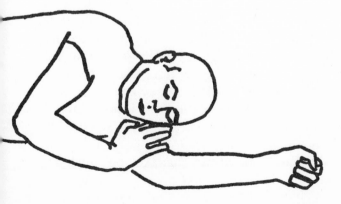

small movements with the fingers and toes, the lips and the jaw.

Some studies have shown that an individual may adopt as many as a dozen different positions in the course of the night. Many of these positions are mirror images of others, however—in terms of psychological meaning, two mirrored positions are much the same. Also, many positions are assumed only for a short time, and are in essence merely transitional or interim positions. For example, the individual may pause while shifting from the semi-fetal to the royal position, so that the upper part of his back is already flat on the bed while his hips and legs remain partially turned to one side. It is as though the person were suddenly "frozen" midway between one position and another. An explanation for this phenomenon, it seems to me, lies in the nature of REM sleep. A person may initiate a shift in position, but be unable to carry it through because of the paralysis that sets in with the start of a dream. Thus these interim positions would not have any special significance when they are of short duration—their basis being physical rather than psychological. A twisted position that is preferred and therefore assumed for long periods of time, becoming a habitual sleep position, is of course important. Such exotic positions will be discussed in Chapter Six.

Subtracting the mirror image and transitional positions, most of us assume only two or three behaviorally meaningful positions during the night. Each of us has a basic individual range of bodily expression, reflecting both our standard discrete defenses and characterological defenses, that we use night after night in a recurring pattern, and which we know to be typical of ourselves. We can, of course, learn a new sleeping position—if we suffer a back injury, for instance, we may have to change our sleep position in order to facilitate our recovery. But a preferred sleep position is stubbornly clung to. We will not change that position unless we change our life.

People who usually live in the city sometimes report that they assume a different sleep position when on vacation in the country or at the seashore. If we feel more relaxed than we usually do—or more anxious—the posture we assume in the sleep world will reflect those feelings. Sleep positions— both the twilight zone alpha position and the omega position of full sleep—exquisitely reflect the immediate life situation. If we change our way of looking at and living in the world, in the course of psychotherapy for example, our sleeping positions will change to express this new behavioral perspective.

The complexities of human character are fully reflected in the number of positions a given person may take in the course of the night, and the particular combination he chooses. One person may, for instance, assume the royal position when first getting into bed. As he drifts off into the sleep universe, he usually abandons this alpha position for an omega position that finds him lying on his side. In interpreting such a change, it could be presumed that this person thinks of himself as the ruler of his existence; his opinion of himself is shown by his choice of the royal position. But then, once asleep, his basic way of meeting life shows itself. In his sleep, no longer feeling it necessary to present a particular face to the world, he demonstrates that he is fundamentally a sensible take-things-as-they-come kind of person. If he spends most of the night in this semi-fetal position, then it can be concluded that it reflects his most basic mode of relating to his world situation. The alpha position that he took on first getting into bed, lying on his back, represents another aspect of his personality, but not his basic orientation.

When a person has difficulty falling asleep, he may change from the alpha to the omega position before sleep. Feeling vulnerable to the anxiety or stress that is keeping him awake, he may find himself unable to enter the sleep world in his customary position. Drawing upon additional character defenses to ease his anxiety, he will assume a position offering a greater sense of security or command of the bed-space. Or the individual may assume a position that is quite different from both the alpha and omega positions he would normally adopt. This was the case with a patient of mine, a young woman who led a very loosely structured, "hippie" kind of existence, taking on a variety of temporary jobs and moving from one short-term personal relationship to another. When she had a job or was involved in a relationship she usually began the night on her side and then changed to a prone position. But when her life situation became more stressful, through the loss of a job or the breakup of a relationship, she found it impossible to sleep unless she assumed a full-fetal position. Only that position afforded her the degree of security necessary for entry into the sleep world at these times.

Although most people have a range of sleep positions—expressing the basic stances that they take in life—it should be clear that some combinations are more likely than others. A person who usually sleeps in the royal position is unlikely to assume the prone position with any regularity, as an equally preferred position. On Sunday morning, wanting to sleep late but disturbed by a loud phonograph in the apartment above, a royal sleeper might turn over on his stomach, as though to say, "This is my bed and I'm going to stay in it; I'm not ready to get up yet." But on getting back to sleep, the person would probably return to the royal position—the one that expresses his basic way of living in the world.

The reader should not assume that one position is necessarily "better" than another, nor should there be concern that a given sleep position reveals a person as "abnormal." Someone who sleeps in the royal position may, despite his overall confidence, at some point encounter difficulties in coping with his life that make it necessary for him to seek therapy, while someone who sleeps in the full-fetal position may never experience a threatening stress that requires treatment or special attention.

Moreover, while the sleep positions have definite meanings, a simplistic approach to the material should be avoided. The four most common positions discussed in this chapter constitute only an introduction to the full story of sleep positions. In subsequent chapters, as we deal with small parts of the body, exotic positions and couple sleep, a more complete vocabulary of the expressive range of sleep positions will be developed.

We first begin to develop a definite sleep position at the age of about three months. The infant, who now has the capacity to begin moving freely and to turn over by itself, starts to assume a favorite position. This occurs at the time the NREM-REM sleeping cycle, with its built-in security, becomes fully available to the child. During childhood, beginning to act out life's drama, there may be experimentation with a variety of sleeping positions, some of them quite peculiar. Some children, for example, may go through a period in which they lie facedown with the body weight supported by the knees and their backs in the air. This position, called the *Sphinx,* shows a strong resistance to the sleep world, and can be seen in children who resent being put to bed at a particular hour.

It is indicated that the child assumes a definitive sleep position at about the age of seven—by which time the major character profile to be assumed by the individual in life is more or less laid out. Changes in sleep position sometimes occur during puberty, reflecting the turbulent events of this critical growth period. The daughter of a friend, a basically healthy girl of twelve who had been the victim of a minor sexual incident, sent me the following letter about her change in sleep positions:

"I just read your article about sleeping and flipped my

lid. You see, about two years ago I was a 'semi-fetal' sleeper. At first I slept on both sides, switching back and forth (it gets boring sleeping on one side). Then I got tired of switching back and forth so I picked the most comfortable side, the right side. Now I'm a 'prone' sleeper. I never sleep on the side of the bed. Always the middle. And I do like to organize everything around me. I just wanted you to know."

Although the girl herself was unaware of why she had changed her position, it clearly reflects her defensive re- action to being molested. The choice of the prone position demonstrates a desire to achieve greater security in her sleep world and control over her adolescent emotions. Possibly, as she matures and the memory of her ordeal becomes less intense, the need for guarding herself will lessen—in which case she may once again return to her semi-fetal position. In fact, the sleep position does not seem to become finally fixed until the age of eighteen or nineteen, when the average young person lives away from home for the first time, and begins the break from childhood dependency.

As noted, we can change our sleep position in later life. Frequently this occurs in response to physical need, because of illness or injury. Some cardiac patients like to sleep more or less sitting up, using a number of pillows to support the back. As the heart becomes less and less able to do its work, greater numbers of pillows are used. Such cardiac patients find themselves unable to assume the horizontal position normally associated with entry into the sleep world—they feel that their very existence, limited by difficulties of circulation, needs propping up.

Back problems and injuries are perhaps the most common reason for advising a change in sleep position. One patient of mine, who preferred to sleep on her stomach, developed a back problem that made it necessary for her to sleep flat on her back. She adjusted to the change in the following way: lying on her back toward the left-hand edge of the bed, she would hook her left heel under the side of the mattress and her right heel under the foot of the mattress; her left arm, extended over the edge of the bed, also gripped the underside of the mattress, while the right arm was thrown fully across the top of the bed grasping the top. In this way she was still able to command her sleep world as fully as she had when she slept in the prone position, giving her the security to be able to fall asleep.

Individuals who sleep in the prone position with their arms extended over their heads run the risk of developing the brachialplexus syndrome, in which the nerves and blood vessels of the arms become constricted because of excessive muscle tension. In order to relieve the tingling and pain in the arms, a new sleep position must be adopted. Again, this is often difficult to accomplish, since the habitual sleep position is a concomitant of character and of the person's psychological defenses. To adopt a new position is, in one sense, to go against the individual's own nature. The fact that it often takes a long struggle to change positions in such cases shows how deeply ingrained our sleep positions are.

The neurologist Dr. Thorner noted that patients who were forced to sleep in an unaccustomed position in order to mitigate bodily pain would revert to their preferred position as soon as the pain was eased. For example, a patient with liver problems normally slept on his right side. His liver pain, however, made it more comfortable to sleep on his back. When he was given morphine, and the pain disappeared, he slept once again on his right side.

It used to be thought that all sleep movement was caused by simple physical discomfort. Doctors and researchers believed that cramped muscles, or pressure on a given nerve, created the stimulus for the night movement of the body. My own studies, however, have clearly shown that this is not the case. The fact that even individuals suffering from physical pain find it difficult to sleep in what is *physically* a more comfortable—but *psychologically* less secure—new position illustrates the extent to which sleep positions are related to personality rather than bodily comfort. In addition, when people do shift position in their sleep, they often assume a mirror image of the previous position—like a switch-hitter in baseball—rather than a basically different configuration. Physical discomfort no doubt plays some part in the night movements of the body, but the primary influence over the choice of a new position is a psychological one. Whatever position the individual chooses as he moves in the night, it will continue to reflect his unique ways of living in the world, and the psychological defenses he has developed for dealing with his special life trajectory.

CHAPTER
V

SMALL PARTS

THE LANGUAGE OF THE BODY in the dark can be simple or complex. Like a written sentence, the basic position provides a fundamental structure of meaning, but one that can be heightened or modified by the placement of the hands and feet, as well as other small parts of the body. Like the adjectives and adverbs used to give a simple sentence additional color and significance, the small parts of the body often suggest a more intricate meaning—even to the point of giving an entirely different tone to the basic position that is assumed. These small parts are also used expressively to indicate a person's relationship to the bed-space and to other people, giving further demonstration of the individual's way of living in the world.

The hands and feet are the most important of the small parts of the body. The heels, ankles, wrists and elbows can be used in many ways to express personality. The calves, knees and thighs also have their story to tell. Even the buttocks can be expressive, when two people sleep together in the same bed.

Let us begin with the feet.

In the day world we stand upon our feet. Our legs carry us forward through life, whether we shuffle, amble, walk or run. During an analytic hour, many patients keep one foot on the floor as though to get a running start off the couch when faced with an anxiety-provoking thought or feeling. In sleep, too, the positioning of the feet tells much about how the individual stands in life, and how he moves forward. A 1944 study showed that many people use their feet to grasp the bed. People who resist change in their lives, who are wary of the unknown or unexpected, often hook one or both of their feet beneath the mattress, like the woman discussed in the previous chapter. When sleeping with a partner, some people will wrap their feet around the other person's legs, as though trying to keep in step with the partner's own movement through life. Conversely, a person may hang his feet loosely over the side or foot of the bed—

showing a refusal to commit himself fully to its topography. Like the patients who keep one foot on the floor when lying on the analytic couch, these people show a need to have an escape route available to them at all times.

Crossed ankles also have their particular meaning in the vocabulary of body language. This meaning was revealed to me one day by a patient. Asked to assume the position in which he slept, he lay down in a semi-fetal position and said, "You see, I'm perfectly normal." He knew, in fact, that the semi-fetal was the most common of all sleep positions. But his ankles gave him away. He slept with his knees apart and his ankles crossed in what I call the *Chain-Gang* position.

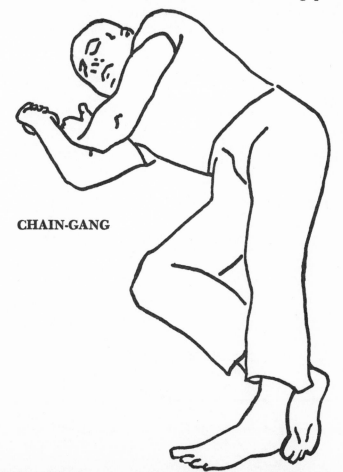

CHAIN-GANG

This description gives an exact picture of this patient's problems in dealing with his life. He was hobbled in his personal relationships, unable to move forward into a meaningful degree of intimacy with a woman—any relationship that he entered into had a high intensity at first, but because of his fear of real involvement he would soon fall by the wayside. In addition, when he began treatment, he complained of boredom at his job, an inability to complete his final thesis, and a high degree of personal immobility in many areas. In spite of the fact that he appeared quite proficient and accomplished, with two separate fields of specialization in his educational and professional background, he found himself a prisoner of his own anxieties, unable to achieve a sense of mobility. The position of his ankles in sleep reflected his difficulties exactly.

SANDWICH

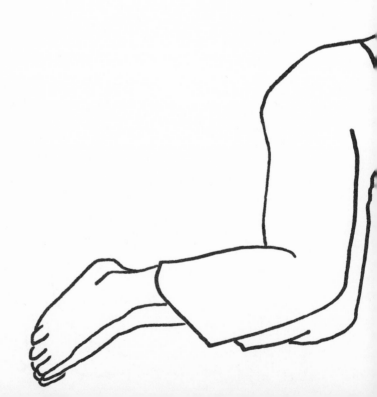

There are several other configurations of the legs that are of significance when sleeping on one's side. Many people who sleep in the semi-fetal position place the legs precisely on top of one another, the thigh, knee and ankle of one leg hewing to that of the other. I call this the *Sandwich* position, and it is indicative of a considerable degree of conformity in the person's life. In the day world, as in sleep, such people seek out a symmetrical relationship with the world; they avoid as much as possible any deviation from what other people expect of them, keeping themselves in line.

Some individuals, although they sleep on their sides, stretch their legs straight out, breaking the usual semi-fetal configuration. Some months ago a television news crew came to my office to film a feature story about my work on sleep

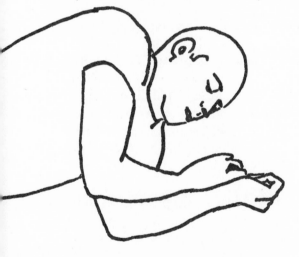

positions. The news reporter spontaneously lay down on my couch to show me the position in which he slept. Lying on his side, he extended his legs fully toward the bottom of the couch, one leg on top of the other. I interpreted this position as showing a high degree of activity—the reporter would not allow himself to relax completely even in sleep, but kept himself prepared to step straight back into the stand-up day world. I call this the *Hero* position. An extension of the Sandwich position, the Hero indicates an active and assertive personality, typical of someone who is always on the go—as, indeed, the reporter had to be in his chosen profession.

Another variation of the semi-fetal position, again involving the lower extremities, is the *Flamingo*. Here, the person has one leg straight out, while the other leg is bent at the knee and flexed at a sharp angle, sometimes with the foot tucked under or over the upper calf of the straight leg. The straight leg shows the individual's assertiveness—but the flexed leg shows relaxation and passivity. This position is characteristic of persons commonly referred to as being passive-aggressive in their personalities. In their relationships, such people show both passive and aggressive attitudes, with both elements as strong parts of their character. Life may well become a kind of tennis match between these two aspects of the personality, with first one side and then the other scoring a point.

The position of the upper legs in sleep is a good indicator of sexual openness—or its reverse. When the thighs are apart in the *Wedge* position, leaving the way open to the genitals, the individual is generally open and giving in his or her sexual relations. When the thighs are kept tightly together in the *Clothespin* position, timidity, repression and defensiveness in the sexual area are indicated. In the chapter on couple sleep, we shall be dealing much more fully with the sexual implications of various positions, and with the use of the genitals, the buttocks and the breasts in establishing

FLAMINGO

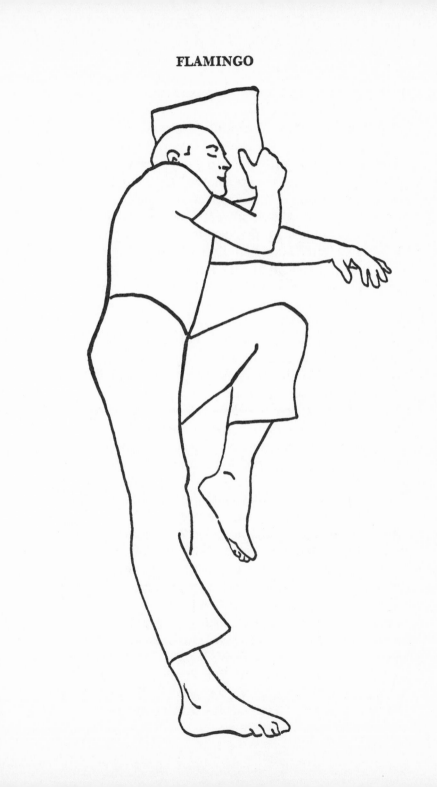

libidinous contact with the sleep partner.

The hands are for touching. They are for grasping or holding on to things. We can also make a fist with our hands. The way we hold our hands can show tension or relaxation. Just as an orchestral conductor uses his hands to communicate to the musicians the character and emotion inherent in the notes of a symphonic score, so too we use our hands, in the sleep world as in the day world, to express the rich melodies of our individual lives. Some of us use gestures more than others—in Mediterranean lands the use of the hands is an art form in itself—but however we may hold or use them, they convey our feelings about ourselves and the world we live in.

Many people use the hands to hold on to the the bedpost or some other part of the bed when they sleep. I call this the *Umbilical* position. Such people need to hold on to someone or something in life, and are often clinging, essentially dependent personalities—they have not allowed themselves the freedom to let go and be themselves. Yet it should not be forgotten that we have two hands. And it may often seem that the right hand doesn't know what the left hand is doing.

For instance, a man may clutch the bedpost with his right hand. But the left hand will be stretched out over the edge of the bed, hanging loose in space. The loose hand indicates that the man is unwilling to fully commit himself to the geography of the bed—or to his life environment. The dependency shown by the clutching right hand is contradicted by the loosely suspended left hand. In this case, we have an individual with a strong element of dependency in his personality, but who nevertheless refuses to surrender himself entirely to this need. With his hands, he demonstrates the extent of his ambivalence. This conflict between his need to hold on and his need to stay loose will most likely also exist in his waking relationships with other people. He will be uneasy if he does not have someone to cling to—but equally disturbed if that other person demands too much from him emotionally.

Such an interpretation may seem to be giving a great deal of weight to small details. Can the hands really express so much about a person? The answer is yes. Over and over again, through years of observation, I have found that such details of sleep posture reflect the whole person. If a man or woman sleeps in a certain way, habitually, night after night, it is an embodiment of his or her psychological needs and fears. And while the language of the small parts of the body may be quite subtle, it is no less telling.

Particular placements of the hands seem to be generally correlated with the different basic sleep positions. Holding the hands in front of the body, in the area of the upper chest, appears to be an entirely natural placing while sleeping in the typical semi-fetal side position. The most frequent hand position for those who lie on their backs in the royal position is to keep the hands on the mattress at their sides, with the palms curled in a display of maximum receptiveness. In connection with the prone position, it is common for the hands to be extended above the head, with the arms flexed. This *Frog* position has the disadvantage of sometimes causing circulatory problems in the arms—the brachialplexus syndrome mentioned earlier.

If the hands are tightly interlaced, holding in the stomach, or layered one on top of the other across the stomach, a new meaning is acquired. This is a protective position. The stomach is, of course, associated with food, and has close connections with the mother-child feeding relationship. A female patient who had been a battered child slept in the royal position with her hands layered on her stomach. Her mother, often disturbed and drunk, would beat her sleeping child on the abdomen. In this case, the daughter assumed the royal position not because of the usual reasons of security and openness, but so as to have maximum alertness against the possibility of attack while she slept. The layering of the hands indicates that she did not in fact feel secure in this position—if she had been secure the hands would have been relaxed, corroborating the openness of the basic position. In therapy, as she improved, this patient began to sleep in a side position, showing conclusively that the royal position was not "natural" to her but rather assumed as a physical defense. At one point, when the therapist went on vacation and the patient was deprived of the security she had gained from the treatment relationship, she reverted to sleeping on her back with her hands layered across her stomach. Once the analyst had returned, she spontaneously assumed the side position again.

The extension of the hands above the head in various positions can also be significant. We have previously mentioned the *Water-Wings* position, in which the head rests in

WATER-WINGS

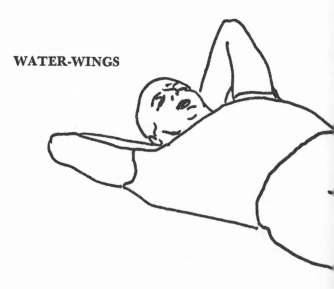

the palms of the hands with the elbows extended on either side—characteristic of individuals who use intellectualization as a defense, funneling all sensations into the head. In eulogizing the late social philosopher Hannah Arendt, novelist Mary McCarthy said that Miss Arendt was the only person she had ever *seen* think—and went on to give a description of Miss Arendt lying on a couch with her hands in the Water-Wings position.

In the *Gymnast* position, the person lies on his back with his hands held a few inches out from the side of the head at ear level, as though he were lifting weights or chinning himself on a bar. This placing of the hands intensifies the sense of self-satisfaction associated with the royal position. Sometimes, however, the hands are extended fully over the head in the *Surrender* position, almost as if the sleeper were obeying the command "hands up." Here, the hands are out of

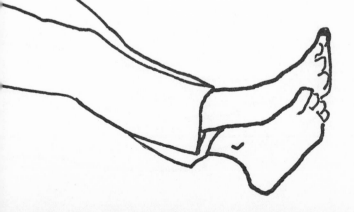

action and highly visible, indicating a passivity that to some extent contradicts the basic royal position—as we all know, there are weak kings as well as strong ones.

Sometimes in sleep the hands are used to grasp the opposite shoulder. This may be done with one hand or both. It is as though such people were cold and needed the warmth of someone else, or to hold themselves together. Yet people who adopt the *Huddle* position are seldom truly open about their need—the fingers are usually held tightly together, rather than spread out as they would be in a true embrace.

In waking life we explain a great deal with hand gestures, miming what we want to say. In sleep, unable to communicate our thoughts in terms of coherent speech, our hands can become even more articulate—like a deaf-mute, we use them in highly expressive ways. One man, for instance, always slept with one finger upright across his mouth, exactly as though he were saying, "Shh, be quiet." Another of my patients slept with her hand covering the genital area— a gesture simple enough to interpret. But in this case there was a contradictory element to this protective gesture. Sometimes, this woman would fall asleep with a packet of matches in her hand, with the hand placed as usual over her genitals.

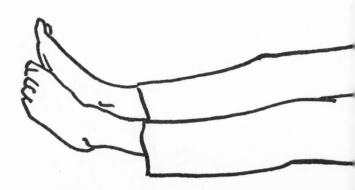

This showed her potentiality for fiery sexual arousal—while at the same time she protected herself against it.

When the hands are balled up into fists, in the *Boxer* position, aggressiveness and hostility are vividly demonstrated. A young man who usually sleeps with his hands open, but makes them into fists when he visits his parents is very clearly indicating how he feels about his family. As we shall see in the chapter on couple sleep, the hands and other small parts of the body are often used to show aggressiveness toward and love for the sleeping partner.

One patient of mine, a divorced woman, learned to her surprise that her former husband was about to marry one of her best friends. Her reaction to the news, in her sleep world, was to hold her hands in a fist-like configuration, but with the thumb buried inside the hand between the palm and the other fingers. This mock fist showed her ambivalence toward her own aggressiveness. In waking life, she handled the situation in exactly the same manner, experiencing resentment and anger, yet at the same time being unable to express it because she felt that she had no objective right to be angry.

A woman with cancer, who had her right breast removed,

BOXER

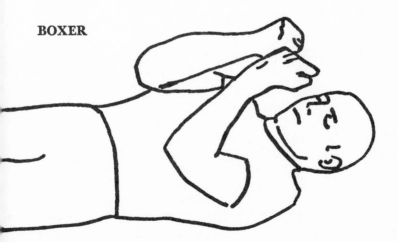

changed her sleeping position in two ways. Previously, she had slept primarily on her right side, but following the operation she shifted to the left side for greater physical comfort. To express the psychological pain she felt, she began sleeping with her face buried in her hands—a classic gesture of mourning.

All these examples show how profoundly mimetic the hands can be in the sleep world. In sleep we act out the dramas of our lives, using our bodies instead of our speech to express our joys and griefs, our loves and hates. In the night world, each of us becomes the pantomimist of his own personal saga.

CHAPTER
VI

EXOTIC POSITIONS

THE EXOTIC POSITIONS to be described in this chapter give further demonstration of the degree to which sleep positions disclose the basic ways in which the individual relates to other people and to life situations. Some of these exotic positions are rare, even unique. Others, while more common, are in one way or another extreme—they exceed in the vividness of their bodily expression the positions already described.

One of the most frequently observed exotic positions is the *Ostrich*. Those who habitually sleep in this position, with a pillow over their heads, are obviously trying to shut out the troubles of their lives. They are expressing a desire to ignore the thinking day world as completely as possible, in the hopes that it will simply go away. The aspect of this position that makes it extreme is the fact that the ears are covered.

The ears, after all, serve as our early warning system in the darkness of the sleep world. The auditory sense not only remains the most acute of any while we sleep—it actually intensifies, especially during the REM stages. During waking existence, we can hear sounds in the range between about 35 and 130 decibels, the decibel being the unit used to measure the differences in sound intensity. A conversation at a distance of twelve feet registers 50 decibels, thunder 70, New York City traffic 80 or more; the 130 upper limit marks the loudest noise that the human ear can stand—a level approached by the amplified sound of some rock groups at their concerts.

In sleep, however, the lower limit is extended, and the ear becomes sensitive to sounds that it would not ordinarily pick up when we are awake. As noted before, though, we are selective about what we hear when asleep. A person living next to an elevated railway will screen out that metallic roaring, yet waken instantly at the small sound of someone fiddling with the front door lock. We are deaf to ordinary sounds, but alert to unusual ones, especially those of danger. The importance of keeping this channel of perception open during sleep, as a matter of self-protection, is emphasized by the fact that I have never found anyone who usually sleeps with his hands holding on to or covering his ears. Thus, people who cover their heads with a pillow for the greater part of the night, muffling their ears, are indicating very strongly that they want to filter out the demands of waking existence. (The use of ear-plugs has a similar psychological significance.) It is more important to such people to bury their heads in the sands of night than to guard themselves against possible danger.

A related position is the *Mummy*, in which the person swaddles himself so completely in the bedclothes that he is virtually trussed up for the night. The covers will be pulled up over the head as well. These individuals are hiding from the world, giving a graphic demonstration of their timidity. Just as they fear confrontation with the day world, and tend to withdraw to a corner of the room at a party, so too they attempt to withdraw and hide in the night world. Like the Envelope Man previously discussed who always placed cigarettes, matches, a glass and a bottle of Coke on his bedside table for security, people who assume the Mummy position often show a need to have certain objects important in waking life close at hand during the night—much as the Egyptian pharaohs required that their treasures be buried with them as they embarked on their dark voyage across the river of death into the afterworld.

MUMMY

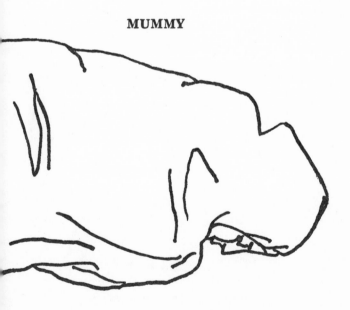

The *Sphinx* position is, as we have seen, most commonly taken by children, but it is not unknown in adults. Crouched on their knees, these people have literally got their backs up, resisting the sleep world. They may be brought to their knees, as sleep tolls the count, but like a champion boxer refuse to surrender completely to the horizontal. Some children remain in this posture for hours before going into a more normal sleep position, or being placed in one by their concerned parents. In adults, the Sphinx position is often associated with poor sleepers, who want to get back to the day world as quickly as possible in order to continue their combat with life.

One of my patients habitually slept in what some of her friends, who had observed her sleeping posture, called the *Monkey* position. She lay with her shoulders pressed back against the bed, while her lower body was turned to the side and somewhat curled up. Her right leg was twisted over the left, protecting the genital zone, with the lower part of the leg somewhat extended. Her other leg was stretched full out, as were her arms, flung upward above her head. The curled trunk and flailing extremities have a characteristically monkey-like appearance.

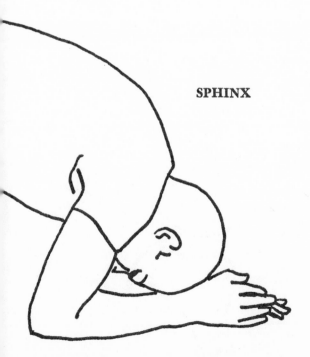

SPHINX

The Monkey position is one of contradictions. The arms and hands are reaching out, as though seeking contact, yet the genitals are guarded by the covering thigh. The upper half of the body seems to be trying to assume the royal position; the lower half, the semi-fetal position. The young woman exhibited similar contradictions in her waking life. She regularly sought sexual contact, but found herself unable to establish open relationships with her partners. She was a person of much feeling, but twisted away from the full expression of it.

The Monkey, or a variant of it, is often assumed briefly in the course of the night by many people as they turn from

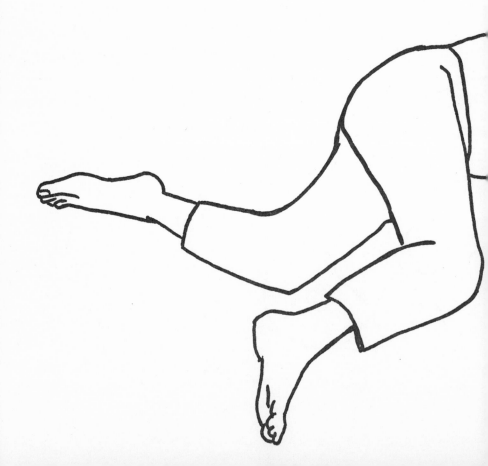

a semi-fetal to a royal position, or vice versa. But when it is merely a transitional position of this sort, its significance can be discounted. It is only when it is adopted as a preferred position for a major part of the night that it should be behaviorally intrepreted.

One patient of mine had had difficulty sleeping since early childhood. Because of whirling thoughts that went racing through his mind, as he attempted to control a fearsome world, he regularly found himself unable to get to sleep. As a result, he would be too fatigued to function at school or on his job the following day. To avoid these problems, he

MONKEY

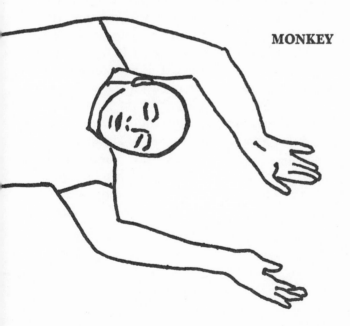

had developed a sleep position that for a time facilitated his entry into the sleep world. He used two pillows, one for his head and the other as a core around which to wrap himself. The core pillow would be pressed against his chest and clasped firmly in his embracing arms, with his body drawn up in a full-fetal position and his right hand placed close to his cheek. When two pillows were unavailable—while traveling, for instance—he would improvise a second pillow from his jacket or raincoat and place this under his head.

He went to a hypnotist for his continuing sleep disturbances, and subsequently began to use a new tactic for getting to sleep. In response to a tape-recorded hypnotic suggestion, on first getting into bed he lay flat on his back with his left hand at his side. But in order to sleep in this position, he found it necessary to use his right arm in a way not suggested by the hypnotist, covering his right eye with it. He stated that he did this in order to shut out part of the world—but at the same time he kept the left eye open on the world in order to distract himself from his racing inner thoughts, until the combination of the prescribed sleeping pills and the suggestive effects of the hypnotic tape message allowed him to fall asleep. I call this position the *Cyclops*. The Cyclops patient could not use a sleep mask because his thoughts would overwhelm him unless he kept his left eye open. It is interesting to note that when drawing projective figures

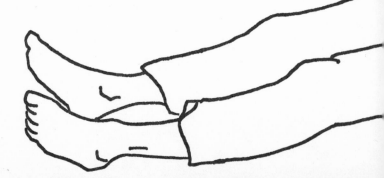

(which represent the self-image on psychological tests), this young man would leave out the pupils of the eyes in both the male and female figures, with only the wide-open outline of the eyes staring out at the world.

At present, after some treatment, this patient has become less anxious, and the world less of a threat to him. As a result, he no longer feels the need to keep one eye open while falling asleep. His whirling thoughts are more under control, and he now uses a sleep mask. And in his alpha position, he now lies on his back with the pillow placed on his chest. As he feels himself falling asleep, he continues to adopt the old full-fetal omega position, wrapping himself around the core pillow. But the fact that he now keeps the pillow on his chest, at the ready for entering his omega position, shows his increased confidence that he will in fact be able to fall asleep. His basic inhibition against the full unfolding of his being, illustrated by the full-fetal posture, continues—but having grown in other aspects of his personality, the exotic Cyclops position is no longer a necessity. Once again, we can see how the sleep position will change if the individual alters his way of living—in this case through psychotherapy.

CYCLOPS

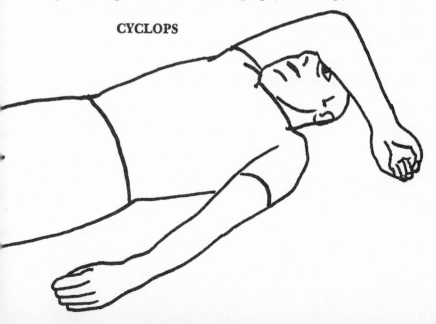

Another unusual position involving a pillow is one that I call the *Dutch Wife*. A Dutch Wife is a long round, bolster-like linen pillow covered by a cotton pillowcase. It is used in the Far East, having originated with Dutch Colonials, and has a double cooling function. Since the linen has a low specific degree of heat, it cools the sleeper, while the cotton pillowcase absorbs sweat. Customarily, it is placed longitudinally in the bed, and the sleeper embraces it as though it were a sleep partner—and thus its name.

One of my patients, who had no knowledge of this custom, nevertheless adopted the Dutch Wife position, although not for its cooling function—in fact quite the opposite. When he entered treatment, one of the patient's primary complaints was of difficulty in relating to women. He stated that he had sucked his thumb until the age of eight. To break himself of this sucking habit, he then began sleeping with his hand under the pillow. He continued to sleep this way until the age of thirteen or fourteen. Then, in response to the developing sexual thrust of puberty, the pillow began to be moved more and more sideways as he slept. The use of the pillow thus changed from having a security function to a love function. By the age of fifteen, he was sleeping completely on top of the pillow, which was placed lengthwise under him, parallel to the long axis of his body. Between the ages of seventeen and eighteen he went through a defensive period of particularly strong alienation from women—

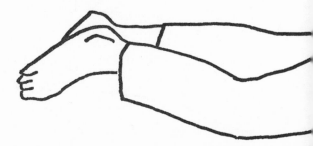

DUTCH WIFE

and so the pillow, which had previously given him comfort by serving as a surrogate love object, was pushed to the floor each night, fully rejected, while he lay in the prone position on the barren bed.

Finally, around twenty, he adopted the Dutch Wife position. He was now more mature and secure, and women began to enter freely into his fantasies. The pillow was placed alongside his body, parallel to it, and he lay with one arm around it. The other arm was extended upward across the bed. He no longer lay prone, but on his left side with his right arm embracing the pillow. This Dutch Wife position allowed him to welcome a fantasy sleep partner into his bed, even though in actual life there was as yet no involvement with a real woman. Later, in discussing couple sleep, we will see what happened to this patient's sleep position after he finally found himself able to develop a relationship with a real woman.

Some people sleep with a pillow between the knees. Often, the rationalization for assuming this position is that, when sleeping in the Sandwich position, pain is caused by the pressure of one knee on top of the other—the pillow is supposedly used to relieve this distressing pressure. This interpretation, as offered by such pillow users, seems superficial. Take, for example, the case of a young woman who began to sleep with a pillow between her knees when she became pregnant shortly after her marriage. Because of the abdomi-

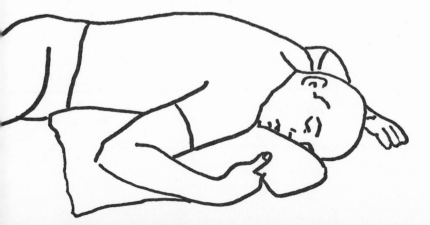

nal enlargement of the pregnancy, she was no longer comfortable sleeping in her preferred prone position, and changed to sleeping on her side. She claimed that without the pillow her knees hurt. But there was more to it than that.

Her personal history reveals that she had been riding horses from a very early age. Her father was an excellent horseman, and began taking her riding with him soon after she was old enough to walk, placing her on the horse in front of him. Later in life, this patient developed into a top-flight rider. During her pregnancy, she felt a special need for security. Thus she assumed the *Equestrian* position in the sleep world—its associations with her father gave her feelings of security and allowed her to face the prospect of giving birth with equanimity. This position proved so satisfying to her that she still retains it, even though her original pregnancy and a subsequent one are long past.

Among the positions recorded by Adler's student Suzanne

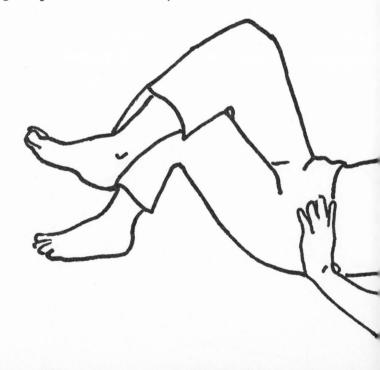

Schalit, there are two exotic positions of particular interest. She describes an eleven-year-old boy who was deeply interested in the theater, and who enjoyed assuming theatrical poses. His theatrics continued through the early stages of sleep. Sometimes he slept on his back with his head held high and both arms crossed behind it; his knees were raised and his legs crossed. I have already pointed out that in my own experience persons associated with the theater commonly sleep in the royal position. In this boy's case, the raised knees and crossed arms create an even more imperial effect than usual. At other times, he would sleep on his side, cheek in hand, his arm supporting his head, while the other arm was placed akimbo on his hip. To all appearances he was striking a nightly pose for a theatrical photographer. I have dubbed this latter position the *Barrymore*. The boy would maintain this gratifyingly flamboyant position for a few hours, and then relax into a more normal sleep position.

An arresting case also described by Schalit is that of a forty-

BARRYMORE

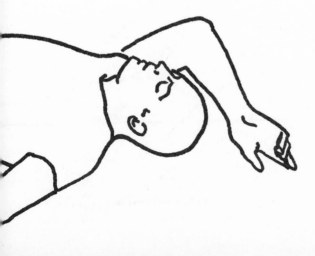

year-old single woman—tall, blond, good-looking—who came from a Prussian military background and who had trained herself to act like the typical Junker. She wore her hair cut short in a military manner, and was always energetic, with everything done promptly and correctly. When she slept, it was always "at attention." Her arms were held straight at her sides. She stretched her head up as far as she could, with her chin tucked in. Even her toes were stretched out as far as possible, in order to achieve a position of maximum General-Staff correctness. I call this position the *Military Brace*, and it is of particular interest to me since one of my own patients slept in a position that echoes it—but with a significant difference.

My own patient, a man in his early thirties, had attended

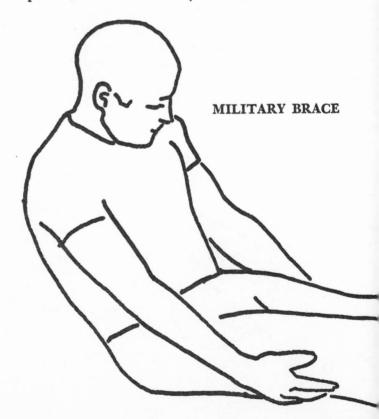

MILITARY BRACE

military school for a large part of his childhood, living in a world of soldier-like training and response. He reported that as a child and also as an adult, he felt overwhelmed and terrorized by a dominating father. He often slept through the entire night sitting up, his hands held at both sides against his body, and his feet extended straight out in front of him. In this case, the upper part of the body assumed the military brace, but by breaking it at the hips, with the upper and lower parts of the body at almost a 90 degree angle to one another, he seemed to be repudiating the obedient, regimented aspects of the basic position. And, indeed, because of his father conflict, there was in his character structure a continual struggle between self-assertiveness and passive obedience to authority —a struggle that made it difficult for him to bring anything to a conclusion or to develop a sense of forward motion in his life.

The fact that his upper body violated the normal horizontal axis of sleep is also of importance. For this patient had many episodes of sleepwalking—most often to raid the icebox and eat everything in it in his hunger for security. And all while he was asleep! After such episodes of sleepwalking— and sleep-eating—he would often return to bed and assume

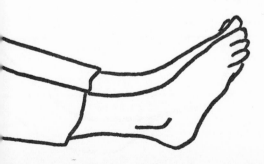

another exotic position. He would sleep on his right side with his head supported on his hand and arm. The arm was bent at the elbow, lifting the upper part of the body approximately 30 degrees from the horizontal plane of the bed. I call this the *Leaner* position. It bears a striking resemblance to the position assumed by Roman sybarites at banquet.

The Leaner position had a double significance in the case of this man. Not only did it mimic a food-eating position, but it can also be viewed as a partial assumption of his broken military brace position. The lounging sybarite and the disciplined soldier marching to orders are clearly at odds with one another as personalities. And so indeed was this young man caught, in waking life as well as in his sleeping positions, between two contradictory aspects of his nature.

To treat this patient for the somnambulism and the sleep-sitting positions—both of which arise out of stage 4 NREM sleep—I prescribed a drug that diminishes stage 4 and facilitates REM sleep, so that instead of walking his conflicts out, he would dream them out instead. The drug worked, and he gave up his extreme sleep positions, but he now complained of stiffness on the right side of the neck. A friend noted that

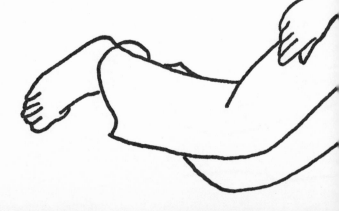

during sleep he would turn his head to the right, arching his body, holding this position almost all night. It was apparent that in his sleep he was still trying to assume the defensive positions which he had previously used but which the drug now eliminated for the most part. It was enough merely to interpret this for him to eliminate even these reduced remnants of his previous disturbed sleep positions.

Several other exotic positions have been reported to me. In some of the following cases I do not have extensive personal knowledge of the individuals involved, and I will deal with them only briefly, suggesting the possible significance of these positions on the basis of what I have learned through my clinical experience.

One such position is the *Matterhorn*. The person lies on his or her back, with one or both knees raised, mountain-like at the center of the bed. As we know, the royal position is an indication of security and self-approval. Yet a raised knee breaks the basic configuration, as well as the horizontal axis. The genitals are considerably more protected in this position than in the usual royal posture. It is as though the in-

LEANER

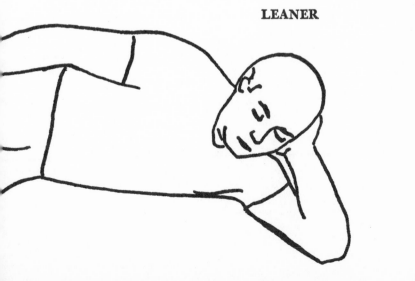

dividual were saying, "I'm a special person, and the way to intimacy with me will not be easy. You must first scale the heights and prove yourself worthy." The sense of self-worth is emphasized here—but the openness, the giving aspects of the royal position, are compromised.

A woman who resisted sexual relations with her husband slept in the *Calisthenic* position—as though her body in the dark were doing sit-ups. She placed pillows behind her back, and slept more or less sitting up, making it impossible for her husband, who slept in a semi-fetal position, to engage her in physical intimacy. Over a number of years she sat up in her sleep farther and farther, withdrawing more and more from her husband. Eventually, she purchased a hassock to support her now fully erect, stiff-backed, defensive sleep posture.

Another woman who slept sitting up did so in quite a different position. Her legs were placed almost in the lotus position, one of the basic configurations of yoga. But instead of leaning back against the pillows, her upper body was bent forward, with her head bowing down over her knees. I call this position the *Clam*. It would seem to indicate a complicated, though not necessarily conflicted, personality. The widespread legs leave the way to the genitals exposed, but, the upper body leans over, giving evidence of protective clamming up and self-absorption.

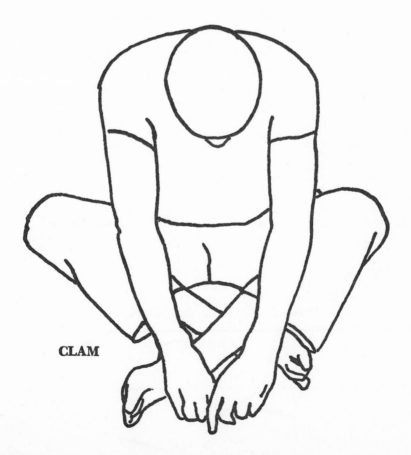

CLAM

One woman slept on her back, fully stretched out, holding the sheet balled up in her left hand near her chin. The other hand was placed above her head, with the palm cupped, facing upward. This *Cat* position is related to the Boxer, the clutched sheet showing her defensiveness. The right hand, instead of being balled into a fist, is partially open, with the fingers apart, as though ready to scratch.

The *Starfish* is an extension of the basic royal position. Here the person lies on the back, but with both the arms and legs spread wide. The self-respecting royal position thus becomes almost self-aggrandizing, showing a need to control the bed-space that is usually associated with the prone position. The *Butterfly*, on the other hand, is a variation of the Sphinx. A young woman who was a dancer by profession reported that she habitually slept in this position, lying prone with her head between her hands, her back lifted slightly into the air, and with her legs spread, wing-like, as though ready

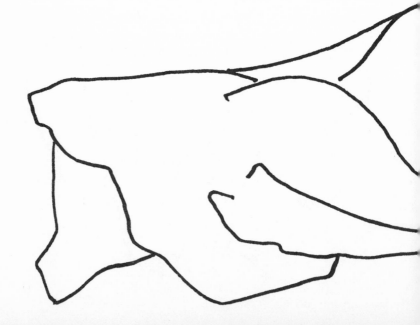

to take flight. The hands, extending like antennae above her head, reflected the seeking nature of her daily life, in which she constantly sought out new people and new professional opportunities.

The *Switch* position is one that I have encountered quite often. In this case, the body in the dark reverses the usual head-on-the-pillow manner of sleeping, and indicates the individual's opposition to a world in which everything is turned around. With the feet on the pillow and the head at the foot of the bed, the topsy-turvy nature of the person's existence is graphically illustrated. This position has special significance in couple sleep, as we shall see in the next chapter.

It is interesting to note, however, that there are cultural and environmental situations in which the Switch position is quite normal. Among the European peasantry both men and women often chose to sleep with their feet on the pillow,

CAT

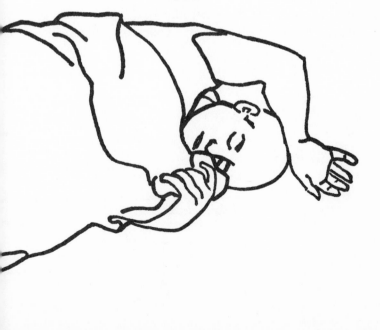

because of a folk belief that their feet did most of the work during their waking lives and therefore deserved the extra comfort of the pillow at night. A 1944 report on American middle-class sleeping habits records the fact that in the days before air-conditioning, many people slept in the Switch position on hot nights because they found it cooler.

One of the rarest of all positions is the *Swastika*. Here, the person lies prone, with one arm extended above the head; the opposite leg is bent at the knee. In all my experience, only two people have reported sleeping in the Swastika—yet physicians and sleep experts generally regard it as the most physically comfortable position that can be assumed in bed. In fact, the majority of advertisements for mattresses show pictures of people sleeping in this position, since it so clearly conveys an impression of relaxation and comfort. The fact that it is so rare in actual practice is one more important indication that the positions in which we choose to sleep reflect our personal ways of living, rather than being dictated merely by physical comfort.

The exotic, contorted and often uncomfortable positions sometimes assumed by the body in the dark give striking visual evidence of the ways of living characteristic of the

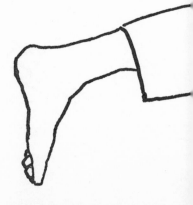

people who choose them. Regardless of physical comfort, the body insistently expresses the whole person—relationships, defenses, conflicts and all. When our lives are bent out of shape, the body in the dark will virtually tie itself into knots in the process of articulating the twists and turns of our existences. And the exotic position will be relinquished—the knots untied—only when the person succeeds in unraveling the personal conflicts that his or her sleep position so eloquently embodies.

SWASTIKA

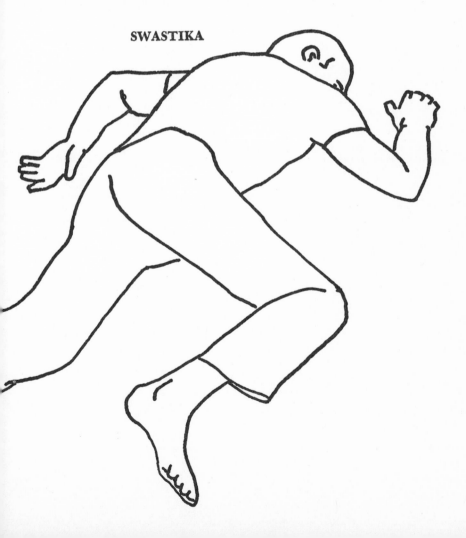

CHAPTER
VII

COUPLE SLEEP

As MY UNDERSTANDING of sleep positions grew, it became increasingly apparent that special sleeping patterns existed in cases where a couple occupied the same bed, that two individuals sharing their lives together gave expression to their feelings about one another in the sleep world. The positions assumed by a person sleeping alone tell one story; but when that person enters into a couple relationship, the preferred sleep position will be affected by the presence in the bed (as in daily living) of another unique individual.

The sleep world is in many ways an extremely private one, yet most of us share our bed-space with another person. Even as we dream our solitary dreams, an arm, a leg, a breast or a buttock will be in comforting contact with the warm body of the husband, wife or lover with whom we travel through our joined existences. Our private, individual experience in the sleep world remains our own, whether we sleep alone or with a partner, but the bodily way in which two sleeping people relate to one another in the bed-space reveals much about the satisfactions and disappointments, the pleasure and trials, of their waking dyadic relationship. Even in sleep we use our bodies to communicate with or express our feelings about our partners.

At the beginning of a relationship between two people, the couple will most frequently assume the so-called *Spoon* position. Both partners will lie on their sides in a semi-fetal position, with their bodies nestling against one another like two spoons in a drawer. Both lie on the same side facing in the same direction, usually with the genitals of the posterior partner pressed against the buttocks of the other. Often the posterior partner holds the anterior one by placing a hand tenderly or possessively on the breast or chest, the stomach, or the genitals. The legs of the couple may be intertwined, showing their desire to merge together. Or one of the legs of the posterior partner may possessively overlie those of the other.

SPOON

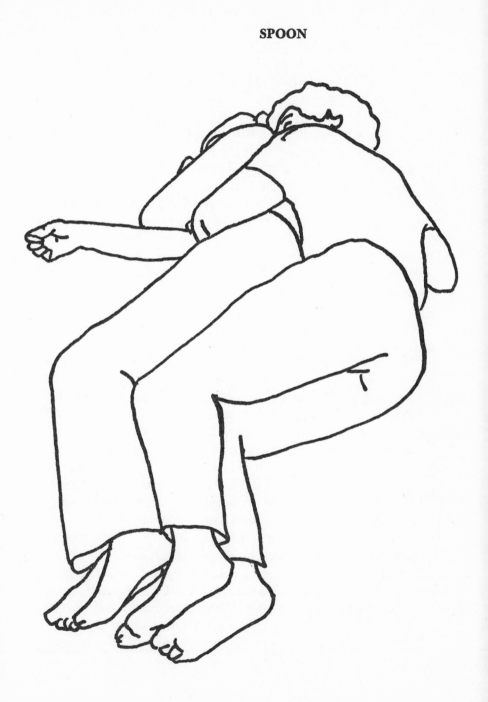

In our society, where the male is dominant, the person assuming the posterior position at the beginning of sleep is usually the man. If the woman lies behind the man, it may indicate a protective or nurturing attitude or simply that the woman is more giving than the man, and lies behind him so that she may more easily embrace him in her sleep. As the night passes, on the slow journey to dawn, it is common for couples to assume a mirror image of the initial Spoon position. As one or both tire of sleeping on one side, they will shift in tandem, without waking. In most cases, regardless of who begins the shift to a new position, the other partner will follow suit synchronously, the couple performing a graceful nocturnal pavane.

The Spoon position makes possible maximum physical and emotional intimacy during sleep, and often involves marked erotic overtones. The quality of sexual intimacy and openness between the couple may be expressed by the placement of the arms and hands. When the posterior partner habitually places a hand upon the genitals of the other, a particularly intense sexual relationship is clearly demonstrated. Sometimes this hand position eventually involves a certain amount of masturbatory stroking in the course of the night—especially in conjunction with a REM period, with its characteristic genital tumescence. This "foreplay," beginning while the couple are still adrift in sleep, may gradually bring on arousal, waking the partners and initiating sex.

Tenderness of feeling may be expressed by the way in which a hand cups the breasts. To place a hand across the stomach of the partner is obviously a more neutral positioning; the encircling arm maintains the closeness of the embrace, but the hand itself avoids contact with the more overtly sexual areas.

The *Hug*, a position that is sometimes assumed by couples who are extremely in love, is the ultimate position of bodily intimacy in sleep. The partners lie on their sides, front-to-front and face-to-face, with their arms tightly clasping one another, as though to fuse themselves into one being.

Although the Hug is not as common as the Spoon, it frequently occurs at the beginning of an intense relationship, and in rare cases is maintained over the years. I recently attended a family party at which a cousin and her husband came over to tell me about their mode of couple sleep. They had been married for decades, and throughout their forty years together, they had always slept face-to-face, holding one another—and they still continued to do so. I immediately shook both their hands and congratulated them on the enduring closeness of their marriage!

My congratulations were in order because in most marriages, or couple arrangements, the partners tend to drift bodily apart, like the continents, with the passage of time, opening a physical gap between them. There is, in fact, a kind of natural history of couple sleep that holds true in most cases. The partners may sleep in the Hug position at the beginning of their marriage. Then after some months, the Spoon will be adopted. After about five years, another change will occur. While still sleeping in the Spoon position, they will no longer be in such close contact with one another. A narrow inlet of clear bed-space will open between them—but some direct contact may be maintained with a touching hand, knee or foot, as though a connecting emotional isthmus remained between the two drifting bodies.

The progression toward greater separateness usually continues over the years. Larger beds are acquired, so that more distance between the partners is possible. This change, which usually comes after about ten years, is often accompanied by a further alteration of the sleep position itself—for it is common at this point to find the two mates sleeping with their backs to one another, while still lying on their sides. Some remnant of tender contact may be maintained, usually with the feet. Or one of the partners may adopt a basically preferred position, such as sleeping prone, that he or she had avoided in the early years of marriage because it reduced physical intimacy.

After fifteen years together, a further step may be the use of a Hollywood bed, with two individual mattresses, individual sets of sheets and blankets, and joint contact between the partners delegated to the common headboard. Twin beds are sometimes used, with a lamp stand in between. Finally, if they have the luxury of space, the couple may sleep in separate bedrooms, sharing a common bathroom, the doors open on either side. Then, it is only when the libidinal fires burn high that they will find the way to one another in the night.

It is important to understand that this progression toward physical separation, with a continual lessening of bodily contact during sleep, does not necessarily mean that there is any emotional rift between the couple. It generally means simply that the couple have achieved so much mutual security, in terms of their enduring relationship, that they can tolerate physical separation during sleep without feeling a corresponding sense of emotional alienation. Physical contact and emotional communication are not, after all, the same thing. In a crowded elevator, for instance, there is a maximum of physical contact and a minimum of emotional exchange. In a long-lasting couple relationship, there can be a maximum of shared emotional response and closeness, even though the two partners sleep in separate bedrooms. In such marriages, of course, physical intimacy continues to be expressed, but primarily through actual love play and coitus.

On the other hand, there are cases in which the decline of sleep intimacy can be a sign of emotional schism as well, of the diminution or even the dissolution of love and mutual caring. For instance, if one or the other of the partners begins to draw away into an isolated corner of the bed shortly after a marriage begins, it may signal a withdrawal of love. Normally, at this point the desire and need for physical communication would be at its most potent, since physical and emotional closeness are most affectionately intertwined during the early years of a couple relationship.

Similarly, if there is an abrupt or drastic change in the sleep relationship of the couple—at whatever point in time—it inevitably reflects an equally sudden change in their waking relationship. A man who has slept in the Spoon position, in close contact with his wife, for the first three years of their marriage, but suddenly begins sleeping on the far side of the bed with his back to her, night after night, is telling her that he is drawing away from her in their life as a whole. This kind of change, which I call the *freeze maneuver*, graphically states, "Stay away from me." No longer do the couple move in tandem in the night; each of the partners occupies his or her own individual territory in the bed-space. Sometimes the rejected partner will try to move closer to the other, attempting to thaw out the freeze and reestablish contact. In the next chapter, "Sleep Love and Sleep Hate," we will see what happens when one person "reaches" out to the other in the sleep world, trying to reunite their sundered territories.

The sudden use of the freeze maneuver contrasts greatly with the normal graduated progression toward greater separateness in the sleep world, as we would expect to find it in a healthy marriage. Such drawing apart is usually a slow process. After a few years of marriage, a couple might adopt the Spoon as an alpha position, and then, once they feel themselves falling asleep, turn over into two less closely connected omega positions. The initial Spoon position establishes the sense of mutual security the partners need to fall asleep—while the omega positions give them greater individuality in their actual sleep. At various times during the night journey—particularly in conjunction with the arousal of the recurring REM periods—the couple may move together again.

The degree of sleep intimacy between a couple can also be affected by work schedules and special patterns of daily living. One couple who both work on the production of films find that their sleep relationship changes according to whether they are working. When they are both on the job, they regularly have to get up at 6 A.M., and often must continue working until 10 o'clock at night. During the week, knowing that they have to get up early, and being very tired, they tend to sleep farther apart in the bed than they do on weekends or when not working. At those times, aware that they can sleep as late as they choose, they intertwine to a much greater degree and relax much more fully.

Thus, the natural history of couple sleep is a slowly evolving process. Change does not take place overnight, but over the course of years. And even as new sleep positions are adopted, there will be occasional returns to the former physical closeness. A couple who have been married ten years, and now usually sleep with their backs to one another, may on occasions of special joy assume the Hug as an alpha position, demonstrating the awakened passion of the moment, recreating the romantic feelings of their first years together.

Preferred sleep positions, the habitual characterological positions that each of us has developed by the time we are young adults, are often less in evidence at the beginning of a love relationship or marriage. The wife may normally prefer the royal position—when sleeping alone—while the husband might ordinarily assume the prone position. But at the beginning of their relationship with one another, their emotions and the whole direction of their lives are bound tightly together. Thus, by sleeping in the Spoon position together, they are expressing in the sleep world, in a bodily way, the new orientation of their waking lives. Their bodies cleave to one another in the dark, just as their daily activities, their waking hopes and desires, are newly interwoven.

At various points in the night, however, one or the other may temporarily revert to their basically preferred omega sleep position. And this tendency increases as time passes. As the couple's closeness becomes fully established and less exploratory, as the intensity of their focusing one upon the other decreases, a renewed sense of each partner's individuality is likely to arise—and with it a new need for a degree of privacy in the sleep world. Thus, each partner may begin to express his or her sense of the self in the sleep world by choosing a basically preferred position that does not allow as much contact as the Spoon position.

When a couple begin to sleep in preferred positions other than the Spoon, they keep in touch in more subtle ways, using the small parts. Through such contact, the emotional currents are allowed to flow outward and return directly from one to the other. The hands, of course, are the most direct way of establishing this flow during sleep. In some cases they may be used merely to touch the partner, a single fingertip joining them together: or the hand may be used to grasp some part of the other person's body. When the hands actually grasp, they may be showing possessiveness, demandingness or even aggression—one partner has the other "in hand" as it were. When a hand is placed within the partner's armpit, or between the lower thighs, it may show a need to "hang on," demonstrating dependency and an inability to let go of the other because of separation anxiety.

Often a couple will use some other part of the body to make contact, not wanting to seem as possessive or assertive as the use of the hands would indicate. I have found, in fact, that the lower extremities and the buttocks are very commonly used to establish contact whenever there is a need for indirection. If a timid individual wants to touch the person he or she is sleeping with, the toes, the heels, and the knees will be used. To touch someone with these lower extremities seems more "accidental" than to use the more prehensile hands. The buttocks allow for large surface contact, but their use also involves some degree of indirection, since the contact is not so "pointed."

Most partners are keenly aware of one another's favored omega sleep positions—and often have rather strong feelings about the other's sleep habits. If two people sleep in basically the same position, there are sometimes problems concerning which side of the bed which person is going to sleep on. For example, if both prefer to sleep in a left-sided semi-fetal position at the edge of the bed, with an unobstructed outer view, somebody is going to have to give way and sleep behind the other, or change to the right side and lie on the other side of the bed.

People who sleep with their arms widely spread, whether lying on their backs, their stomachs or their sides, inevitably take up an abnormal amount of the bed-space. Their attempted dominance of the bed—and of their mutual life-space—can lead to trouble unless the partner generously or compliantly tends to assume a more restricted position. Full-fetal sleepers, of course, might be perfectly happy to have their beds and their lives controlled by their mates. But a prone sleeper is not likely to be pleased by a partner's attempted takeover of their sleep world.

The position that seems to arouse the most resentment—

on the part of those who do not sleep in it—is the royal position. A number of patients have reported to me their annoyance at seeing their partners lying beside them on their backs in the night. It is as though they sensed the super-confident and superior body message being conveyed by the royal position. And the irritated reaction seems to be: "What makes you think you're so great?"

Obviously, couples who sleep together before marriage have an opportunity to learn a great deal about their pro-spective mates from the way they behave in the sleep world. This is a subject we will be returning to in a later chapter.

When discord develops between a couple, it is inevitably reflected in the couple sleep position. This is a fact that, while neglected by sleep researchers and sex therapists, has been intuitively understood by many novelists and play-wrights. In *Ulysses,* for instance, James Joyce tells us that Leopold Bloom slept with his head at the foot of the bed and his feet on the pillow, while his wife Molly slept in the normal configuration with her head on the pillow. Bloom's Switch position perfectly expresses his relationship with his wife: at this point, they are traveling through life heading in opposite directions. Indeed, Bloom's own particular jour-ney carries him off into the obsessional, inverted nightmare world of Nighttown, through which he prowls like a tor-mented sleepwalker.

When a person sleeps in the Switch or some other peculiar position, it not only reflects the relationship to the sleep partner but can on its own exacerbate the difficulties of the couple. Like the previously mentioned young woman who slept on the bias, some individuals create special problems for themselves because of their sleep positions. One woman reported that she could fall asleep only on her side in the full-fetal position, with her knees drawn up to her chin and her arms tucked in—but, in addition, she had to have her knees and lower legs pressed against the chest of the man with whom she was sleeping. Only with that adhesive contact, in which she became an almost bud-like appendage of the man, could she get to sleep.

Later, as she began to open up her existence through therapy, she was able to fall asleep in a more normal, semi-extended position, but still facing the man and with her right leg now thrown over his chest. She was still holding on, expressing her possessive need. With continued improvement, she began sleeping in the prone position; finally, as she became more and more independent in her living, she came to choose one of two omega positions, sleeping either on her back, or on her left side in a semi-fetal position.

One male patient of mine was involved in relationships with two successive women over a period of time. When he first entered treatment, he slept in a full-fetal position, curled up in one corner and facing outward. At this time, when sleeping with his current woman friend, he always kept his back to her, as though saying, "Don't bother me, don't touch me." This man's personal history was greatly affected by an extremely overprotective mother, who virtually swallowed him up, both physically and emotionally. She constantly embraced him, clutching him to her—and he did not have the strength to escape her maternal clasp. In order to fend her off somewhat, and to prevent complete absorption by her, he withdrew passively in upon himself. This withdrawal showed in his sleep position and his relationship to the young woman with whom he was sleeping.

As his positive feelings about himself, and his self-assertiveness developed during treatment, he began sleeping in the prone position. He had opened up to the world more, but still felt a strong defensive need to control the situations of his life. As he continued to improve, he began sleeping on his back, showing increasing openness, tolerance for emotional contact, and ability to give of himself. He became interested in having more intimate physical contact during sleep with the young woman with whom he was living. Finally, he reached the stage of having her sleep with her head on his chest and shoulders. This position was evidence of a dramatic change in this originally highly guarded and emotionally armored young man. The relationship with this young woman, however, could not be sustained because of other tensions.

Subsequently, he got himself involved with another woman who ironically turned out to be as self-involved as he himself had once been. They slept on a waterbed to heighten their physical intimacy—but in the sleep world she drew away from him. He wanted her to sleep with her head on his chest, as his previous woman friend had. But in her undeveloped emotional state, she couldn't fall asleep unless she was fetally curled in an upper corner with her back to him and without his touching her. In other words, at this point in her life she was behaving in the sleep world just as the young man had at the beginning of his treatment! Usually, in fact, this woman waited until he was asleep, and then stealthily got up off the waterbed to go sleep in her own bed. The inherent frustrations of this relationship proved too great for the young man, and after a while he broke with her. In the course of his treatment, as he learned to open himself to emotional contact, he had come to understand the significance of sleep positions, and recognized in the woman disturbing echoes of his own former problems.

Another couple, one of whom I was treating, had difficulties in their marriage. At this time of conflict, the husband—

who habitually slept on his stomach—would find himself gradually moving downward, easing himself out of the marital bed. This *crab maneuver* went so far that he would eventually end up at the foot of the bed, flopping on the edge, with the lower half of his body on the floor and only the upper half remaining on the mattress. Sidling like a crab out of the bed-space, he was precisely illustrating what he was doing in his marriage itself. For as the conflicts with his wife increased, and he developed more and more negative feelings about the relationship, he reached the point of entering into an extramarital affair.

The cases outlined above will serve as an introduction to the complicated maneuvers often resorted to by couples as they seek to communicate their feelings about one another in the sleep world. In the next chapter, we will be going into further detail concerning the expression of emotions in sleep—whether they be feelings of love or hate. For both these passionate emotions, as well as other varieties of feeling, are fully delineated by the bodily positions and motions of couples during their sleep.

The natural history of couple sleep continues even when a couple are separated. In a February 1976 interview with *Newsweek,* the comedian George Burns spoke of his thirty-nine-year marriage to the late Gracie Allen: "The last few years Gracie was alive we slept in twin beds because she had a bad heart. I found that after she died I could never get to sleep. Finally, I slipped over into her bed one night and it worked." This story corresponds to what I have found to be a general truth about couple sleep: if one partner is absent, because of divorce, death, or merely a long business trip, the remaining person almost invariably "slips over" into the bed-space previously occupied by the other partner.

The explanation for this behavior is quite simple. When the two partners existed as a couple, they each felt as though they had the strength of two, giving them a special, paired sense of security as they embarked each night on the sleep journey. But with the partner gone, the remaining person feels vulnerable and bereft, and attempts to create a sleep world that restores the previous secure situation. Such restoration may extend beyond the sleep world, of course, with these individuals taking on the mannerisms and even dress styles of the missing person.

One patient of mine shows how profoundly sleep can be affected by uncoupling and the resulting sense of loss. The woman in this case began to become aware, in a dream, that her husband was thinking of leaving her. In her dream, her husband forced her to perch precariously on a peg in a wall. Teetering on the peg, she suddenly found herself unable to retain her insecure hold and began to fall. Immediately after this dream, the woman insisted upon changing places in the bed with her husband. It was as though by taking his side of the bed, she could create a more secure position in relation to him.

Once the actual separation did occur, she continued to sleep on the side of the bed she had usurped from her husband. But another change in her position took place. Formerly, she had slept prone with her head turned toward the window, but now she shifted so that she faced the door, as though waiting for her husband's imminent return. Later, she heard of her estranged husband's relationship with another woman. At this point, my patient began to sleep lying across the middle of the bed—that is, at right angles to the long axis of the bed. Her husband divorced her and made plans to marry the other woman. As the wedding date approached, my patient again changed positions, now assuming the Switch position, with her head at the foot of the bed. Through all these permutations, she continued to sleep prone, but expressing her changing attitudes and defenses by shifting from one area of the bed-space to another.

Thus, we can see that we continue to relate to an absent partner in the sleep world, giving bodily substance to our conflicting feelings about the person, just as we continue to think about the person in waking life long after the actual parting has occurred. As might be expected, it is often not until the lone individual forms a new couple unit, and has a new partner to relate to, that the final emotional vestiges of the previous relationship are fully exorcised from the sleep world.

And then, when the new couple unit is forged, a new cycle will emerge. For each of the two new partners, a fresh historical epoch begins, with its own developmental patterns of sleep as the couple demonstrate in the night the meanings of their relationship.

CHAPTER

VIII

SLEEP LOVE AND
SLEEP HATE

THE COUPLE RELATIONSHIP begins with love.

Most people cannot sleep well in the same bed with another person unless there is some feeling of love between them. To enter the sleep world, to set forth on our nightly voyage, we must have security. Unless we trust the partner with whom we share our bed, that security—which arises not merely out of physical closeness, but out of emotional intimacy as well—will probably be difficult to achieve.

Love in the sleep world is closely associated with sex—an association as old as the human species. Sexual release can be achieved with a stranger, but the fullness of the love experience expresses both desire and tenderness. A couple might affectionately embrace one another throughout the night, even though their overt sexual desire for each other had been fulfilled at bedtime.

Sexuality and sleep are so closely associated, in fact, that many people, both men and women, find it difficult to enter the sleep world unless they have had sex first. Over the years I have encountered many cases in which there was even a compulsive need for sexual intercourse as a sleep prerequisite. This compulsion is found not only among couples, of course. It is very common for lonely or alienated individuals to masturbate before sleep. If a person who has developed a need for some sexual activity as a prerequisite for sleep becomes involved in a couple relationship in which the partner does not share this inclination, difficulties may ensue. For instance, a man for whom sex is a sleep requirement may be more interested in his own release than in satisfying his partner's need, so that the sex becomes a selfish rather than a loving act. When the need originates with one partner alone, the other is often left feeling hung up. If the sex and love relationship between a couple is troubled in any way, and leads to attempted but incomplete sexual release, the resulting feelings of disappointment and frustration can make sleep more difficult to attain.

With younger couples, sexual activity can be so arousing that it is difficult to fall asleep afterward. But older couples often find that lovemaking relaxes them and brings sleep on more easily. Orgastic and emotional release can in fact yield a muscular and hormonal relaxation that facilitates sleep—especially when these physiological effects are combined with a psychological sense of strength and security drawn from unity with the loved one.

Sexual activity practiced within the context of a good relationship can aid sleep in another way. When sexual release has not occurred, the tumescence of the genitals and the pelvic organs that takes place in conjunction with the REM phases is more likely to become so arousing that the individual wakes up. On the other hand, some couples occasionally prefer to initiate a sexual episode in the middle of the night, responding to REM arousal. Couples suffering from minor sexual problems may be able to take advantage of a REM arousal phase to engage in sexual relations at a time of natural excitation, possibly overcoming their difficulties. Such couples, keeping in mind that the REM phases recur at approximately ninety-minute intervals, would be advised to go to sleep at the same time.

The fact that sleep and sex are so linked may, ironically, have something to do with the romantic aura that surrounds the idea of "love in the afternoon." To "sleep" with someone, in the colloquial sense, outside the context of the real sleep world, seems to give many people a sense of extra piquancy. To make love in the full light of day, while the rest of the world works, has a certain clandestine attraction— an appeal that often reflects the reality of the situation in cases of extramarital or otherwise illicit relationships.

When a couple makes love before sleep, the sleep positions they subsequently assume are likely to be especially close—at least in the alpha phase. Many couples who ordinarily would sleep with far less contact, will assume the intimate Hug position, or the Spoon, as they drift off into sleep following sexual activity. Occasionally, couples make love and fall asleep either in the classic *Missionary* position, with the man on top of the woman, or with the woman astride. Because of the discomfort and compromised breathing of the person underneath in these coital positions, the partners are usually forced to adopt more comfortable positions within a short time.

Sexual activity seems to be less common in the morning, as couples emerge from the sleep world. As we have previously seen, mental agility returns more quickly in the morning than does physical coordination. While we mentally forge ahead to begin our involvement with the events of the upcoming day, it takes the body a while to catch up. The mental and physical correspondence that occurs as we prepare for bed at night thus seems more conducive to sexual arousal—at night our whole being is attuned to entering the sleep world and the associations between sex and sleep coalesce at their most intense degree.

Also, simply as a matter of physiology, people tend to be less prepossessing in the morning than when they first get into bed at night. The hair is rumpled after a night in bed, and the face somewhat bloated because of the loss of tonus in the blood vessels during sleep. But, as suggested by the song "A Little Lovin' in the Morning," there are couples who find sex the best of all ways to begin a new day.

No matter how much a couple are in love, difficulties can occur in the relationship—and will be reflected in their sleep patterns. In the sleep world, where the body does the talking, communication between two people takes place in a bodily way. When there is friction between a couple in the waking world, the resulting negative feelings will be expressed by the body in the dark. The body can reflect all degrees of a particular emotion—in the case of conflict, from irritation to anger to outright hate. Hostility may be shown in the way one partner stakes his or her territorial claim to the bedspace at the expense of the other. Or angry rejection may be demonstrated, as one partner withdraws to a narrow wedge of the sleep terrain, guarding it resolutely with a hunched and hostile back—as though the person couldn't stand even the sight of the other.

One couple who came to me for help were indeed very much in love; both had been divorced and both were determined to make this new marriage work. The man was an only child, and had been indulged by both his parents. Although he was basically a healthy, assertive individual, he brought to the couple relationship certain problems that resulted from his indulgent upbringing. He found it difficult to be as giving in his affection as his wife wanted. She, in turn, kept reaching out to him. Her mother and she had been the victims of an irresponsible father, and she felt a strong compensatory need for closeness from her husband, both emotionally and physically.

This couple would generally fall asleep facing one another, each holding the other. After he was asleep, the man would change to a different omega position, turning on his side with his back toward the woman. At this point, she would assume the Spoon position, snuggling up close to her husband with her arm around him. Later, as she fell more deeply asleep, she would turn on her mirror side, and they would spend the rest of the night sleeping back to back, bodies touching in a friendly, relaxed way.

However, the wife at a certain point began to feel that she was reaching out to her husband without getting sufficient attention in return. In the sleep world, reflecting her feelings, she began to "spoon" after her husband, trying to draw closer to him as he slept, and spending more of the night pressed against him in the Spoon position. She wanted to be close to him in order to show her love, and in the hope that he would pay more attention to her. But he misread her signals and began to feel that he was being smothered. He would try to control his anger at this, but his smoldering resentment would sometimes break out in a slashing rage—causing such ugly scenes that she reacted with despair at what seemed to be the inevitable destruction of their marriage. At night they did not even kiss, but would just get into bed and turn their backs icily on one another. It was at this dangerous point that they sought treatment.

After gaining insight into their difficulties, and taking positive steps to heal the breach between them, their relationship demonstrated improvement, in the sleep world as well as in the day world. They have returned to their original sleep pattern, but with a significant alteration. She now understands that the fact that he isn't totally giving doesn't mean he loves her any less. She is now sufficiently reassured so that she "spoons" after him only briefly—and he, on his side, accepts this expression of her need without feeling that she is trying to smother him.

Another case in which one partner reaches out toward the other brings us back to the young man who slept in the Dutch Wife position when living alone. In treatment, this young man overcame his earlier fears about women to the point where he became deeply involved in an intimate couple relationship. But he had not overcome all of his doubts. The problem he faced in this particular relationship was that he didn't know if he "really loved" the woman or not, and was thus unable to allow himself complete affection for her. At that time he had dreams concerning invaders from outer space, whom he saw as the enemy and felt he must fight and conquer. In the course of these dreams he would get hurt, though not seriously, and withdraw to a safe sanctuary.

His dreams directly referred, of course, to the young woman, whom he viewed almost as a stranger from another planet, come to invade his world. It was this situation with which he had to contend. He saw himself as vulnerable to hurt—but because both he and the young woman were in therapy, and because their relationship continued to grow, the wounds he suffered did not penetrate deeply. The sanctuary to which he withdrew was a past position of studied aloofness, from the security of which he could ponder his next steps in the relationship.

He was fortunate that this young woman, his sleep and sex partner, was intensely orgastic. At orgasm, she had the perceptual experience of seeing vivid areas of purple, and would also shout exultantly, maximally demonstrating her extreme pleasure. But along with her vibrant sensual reactions, she brought certain difficulties of her own to the relationship. Having been somewhat neglected while growing up, she was insecure and needed reassurance—which he found hard to give since he was taking only tentative steps himself toward emotional responsiveness. As a demonstration of her need for emotional nurturance, at times of stress the young woman avidly sucked her left thumb in her sleep, usually in the last hours toward morning.

Although the young man's preferred position, when sleeping with this woman, was prone on his stomach, he couldn't sleep in this way if she touched him with her legs. During the night, as she attempted to move closer to him, placing her legs against his, he was forced by the narrowness of the bed to turn on his side with his back to her. Thus the couple spent most of the night in the Spoon position, but with a distance of approximately one and one half feet between them. As might be expected from the personalities involved, she slept behind him. Both his arms and his legs were in the Sandwich position, carefully aligned one atop the other.

Even after he had turned on his side, she would continue to make diplomatic overtures to him, bringing her legs up against the backs of his calves. But the tops of their bodies were drawn apart, forming a triangle of space between them that allowed her room to keep her left hand and thumb, which she occasionally popped into her mouth during the night, near her lips. The more she crowded her legs against him, the more he tried to pull away to his side of the bed. Since he feared being overwhelmed by her inexorable advance on the one hand, and being pushed off the bed on the other, he felt trapped. Eventually, he would stop trying to withdraw, since there was no place to retreat to short of leaving the bed altogether, and would reluctantly allow her to press her legs against his.

In fact, in the relationship as a whole, he has come to accept her more completely. After further treatment, he recently has begun to sleep more comfortably with her, and no longer feels a subjective sense of crowding when she presses against him. He reports that he had never slept in the same bed for an extended period with anyone before, and at first found it strange to share the sleep world with another person. No longer feeling that sense of strangeness, he has begun to sleep more toward the center of the bed— and she, for her part, doesn't press him so hard. In both this case and the previous one, the couples compromised in their sleep-world relationship, each accepting the other's needs more fully, just as they did in their waking lives.

The gamut of sleep-world emotions that a couple can pass through is seen with particular clarity in the case of another of my patients, a woman whose sleep behavior strikingly embodied her changing feelings about her husband. At the beginning of her marriage, she would sometimes wake in the night to find herself fondling, stroking and kissing her husband. She would usually lie in his arms, her body moving as closely as possible to his. But as severe conflicts between them began to emerge and increase, she at first drew away from him and later began to physically attack him while they were asleep. Their marital disturbances reached such intensity that she would frequently kick at him with both feet, like a mule. A fraction of a second before the blow actually struck, she would awaken. Since she was still asleep as the action of her legs was initiated, she was able to say that she hadn't known what she was doing. But, of course, she did know. Her body, in the sleep world, was stating in the most explicit way her true feelings about her husband. On occasion, the blow would be so powerful that it would knock him to the floor. She was literally kicking the husband out of her bed! As might be expected, the structure of their marriage could not long endure this level of disturbance, and a divorce followed.

When one partner is rejecting the other, elaborate maneuvers and stratagems are sometimes instituted to keep that partner at a distance. One woman, who wished to avoid sex with her husband, slept in a fully buttoned housecoat with her arms wrapped around herself. This variation on the Mummy position effectively prevented her husband from attaining even the most fleeting contact with her flesh. Another woman took a more imaginative and less obvious tack. Her husband liked to sleep in the Spoon with his genitals against her buttocks. During the REM phases each night, when he would be sexually aroused, his erect penis would poke against her, waking her up. To protect herself from the intrusion, she claimed to be suffering from hemorrhoids, and told him he was causing her pain each time he had his erection. The couple continued to sleep in the Spoon position, but with the husband being forced to lie at the precise minimal distance that would allow him to have an erection without the phallus actually being able to touch her. This situation is the perfect embodiment of the classic Mike Nichols and Elaine May line about "proximity but no relating."

A more complicated case involves a man who was referred to me for treatment after being arrested. He practiced frottage, or frotteurism, from the French word *frotteur*, meaning to rub. Frotteurism is a fairly common sexual activity in large cities, where people are often crowded impersonally together in small spaces. Men who practice frottage seek out women on the subways during rush hour, or at large public events like parades, and rub their genitals against them. From my patient I learned that such men refer to themselves and one another as "customers," a term of obscure derivation. Many of these frotteurs know one another, and will occasionally get together to discuss their exploits and techniques.

Because of special circumstances in his life history, my patient preferred to approach women from the rear, rubbing his organ against a woman's buttock or the backs of her thighs. He particularly enjoyed placing his penis in the gluteal fold, the cleft between the convexities of the buttocks. Wearing a raincoat or long jacket with the pockets cut, he would reach through from inside the pockets to unzip his trousers and withdraw his penis. (Some of the "customers," he told me, would use a penknife or a razor blade to slit the women's pantyhose.) He himself had developed the skill of surreptitiously raising a woman's skirt and pressing himself against her. During the entire procedure, as he rubbed himself against a woman, he would stare off into space as though lost in thought.

The patient claimed to feel an intense love for the women he used in this way, exemplifying Freud's statement, "Perhaps nowhere does the omnipotence of love show itself more strongly than it does in the aberrations of love." Yet there was an ambivalence to his feelings about these women; his hostility was obvious in his need to "dirty" them by ejaculating on them. Because of his personality problems, he was completely unable to understand why the women themselves could have negative feelings about his practices.

This man had been married for many years. But he had

never had intercourse with his wife, being unable even to visualize vaginal penetration, because this to him seemed negative and disgusting. At the beginning of their marriage, his wife was sexually naive, and allowed him to perform frottage with her. Eventually finding this unsatisfactory, she rejected this sexual pattern. Nevertheless, she accepted the relationship without sex, and they continued to sleep in the same bed. She basically supported him with her income, leaving him unlimited free time to spend in the subways.

The sleep-world relationship of this couple is complex and has certain contradictory aspects. The husband sleeps with his upper body curled into a full-fetal position, but with one arm hanging over the side of the bed. His legs, however, are extended straight out in the Hero position. And his buttocks are pushed against his wife, who sleeps either in a full-fetal or a royal position. In both cases, these positions involve unusual combinations of bodily expression.

Let us look at the husband's position first. The full-fetal coiling of the upper body could be expected—obviously he has not opened himself up to dealing with the adult world in the usual terms. It is unusual, however, for an arm to be extended over the edge of the bed when a person sleeps in a full-fetal position. As was discussed in the chapter on small parts, the extended arm indicates a need to have an "out," to be free to go one's own way. In this case, therefore, the unusual combination of the full-fetal upper body position and the extended arm makes sense: he wants to be free to seek out his numerous but fleeting contacts with other women. The extension of the legs in the Hero position, although on the surface appearing to be a contradiction of the full-fetal upper body posture, shows his readiness to jump back into the day world in whose surging crowds he may pursue the elusive fantasy women of his desires.

His wife's alternation between the full-fetal and the royal position is also unusual. But this combination again has a story to tell. The royal position reflects her sense of self-importance in being the breadwinner, and her pride in maintaining the relationship with her husband. The full-fetal position shows, however, that she has in other ways failed to open up fully to life—indeed, she has been prevented from doing so by her husband's problems.

There is a further dimension to this couple history. Although he sleeps with his buttocks against his wife's body, my patient will not tolerate any attempt on her part to unobtrusively initiate contact with him. He must feel that he controls her, and thus any contact between them must be at his initiative. He really does not want to be touched. And this of course reflects his day-world sexual activities, in which he seeks out women in situations where he is the sole active participant in the sexual encounter, the women manipulated and transfixed.

His wife nevertheless does regularly try to make contact with him in the sleep world, placing her feet against his legs. When she does so, he shoves her feet away. Although sometimes when he is not so irritated, he will tickle her feet instead. Since she is ticklish, this is a mild expression of his negativism.

This couple's sleep relationship is an odd one, reflecting a strange marriage. Yet they have remained together for many years, sleeping in the same bed, and within the special structure of their relationship, they appear to be fond of one another.

Kicking the bed partner is the most blatant form of sleep aggression. Some people also flail their hands and arms around in their sleep, and with seeming inadvertence strike out at their partners in the night. Such activity should be distinguished, however, from the thrusting arms and kicking feet that sometimes accompany battle dreams. Battle dreams, which usually occur toward morning, are nightmares that involve the dreamer in a struggle with some monster or force which arouses such terror that he physically strikes back. In most cases, such dreams are not directed at the sleep partner, and the flailing of the limbs should not be taken for an aggressive action but rather a defensive one. Purposeful sleep aggression, on the other hand, is clearly directed at the partner, usually recurring night after night. Often, as we have seen, sleep aggression takes the form of warding off a partner who is trying to draw close in the night.

A male patient of mine, a bachelor in his forties, frightened a woman who was sleeping with him by pounding on his pillow in the middle of the night as though it were a punching bag. In fact, the anger was not directed at her. This man had a history of aggression and extreme pugnaciousness, which, after much effort on his part, had been brought under control. In his early teens his behavior was so explosive, when provoked, that he was referred to a psychiatrist. It was not until he reached his mid-twenties that he was able fully to control himself, by applying his will, by physically turning away from provocative situations, or by polishing his glasses to buy time. His pillow pounding is a remnant of his formerly explosive behavior—but it is always the neutral pillow that is the target in these episodes, and never the sleep partner. Even in his sleep he has learned to control himself enough so that he doesn't hurt the innocent person sharing his bed.

Aside from striking the sleep partner, one of the most common forms of sleep aggression is snoring. There are a number of theories as to why snoring occurs, but we know it takes place in profound NREM sleep, and that the irritating sound is caused by the regular, slow but full inspiration and expiration of air, causing the tonsillar pillars and the soft palate to fluctuate because of the loss of muscle tonus. Occasional snoring, when a person has a cold or has drunk heavily that evening, is not necessarily aggressive. But many patients have reported that when there are particularly strong tensions in the couple relationship, angry partners will snore more often and more loudly. Pathological snoring can be controlled by the use of drugs which eliminate stages 3 and 4 of NREM sleep, or by various mechanical devices. I have sometimes encountered couple relationships in which one partner snores while the other is a very light sleeper, an unfortunate combination. But, paradoxically, exactly the same drug can help with both conditions.

Teeth-grinding (bruxism), flatulating and bed-wetting (enuresis) are sometimes forms of sleep aggression. Nocturnal emissions ("wet dreams") may occasionally be a subtle form of sleep aggression, depriving the partner of the pleasure of mutual orgasm. Nocturnal emissions can also be accusatory, saying in effect, "See what happens when we don't make love?" Both men and women at times furtively masturbate while lying beside a sleeping partner. Like nocturnal emissions, such masturbation may have either an aggressive or an accusatory emotional basis. Even when one partner becomes aware of the other's masturbation, there is usually a reluctance to intrude on something so private by letting on that they realize what is happening.

The couple relationship begins with love—and in the course of the normal, long-lasting marriage, that love is expressed in a variety of ways in the sleep world, usually following the pattern of natural history of couple sleep outlined in the previous chapter. But when a couple relationship founders, withdrawal or aggression will also be embodied in the sleep relationship of the two partners. The emotions of love and hate, and the needs and anxieties that accompany them, are not left behind when we enter the sleep world each night. We carry them with us on our voyage to dawn, and we make them known in the night, telling our partners exactly how we feel about them.

Sometimes, however, the tensions between a couple become so great that they find themselves bereft of the security necessary to entering the sleep world. One partner, or both, will lie awake for hours, obsessively reviewing the problems between them. The person lies in darkness, but is unable to achieve the unity with that darkness that is the basis of sleep. Like millions of other individuals, married and single, the troubled partner becomes the victim of insomnia, wide-awake at three in the morning, alienated from the day world and the sleep world at once.

CHAPTER

WHEN IT'S ALWAYS
THREE O'CLOCK
IN THE MORNING

To INSOMNIACS, "it's always three o'clock in the morning," to use F. Scott Fitzgerald's phrase for "a real dark night of the soul." At that stark hour of the night some insomniacs will not yet have been able to fall asleep, while others will wake to thrash restlessly in the darkness for an hour or more. Insomnia, with its tossings and turnings, its muscular and nervous tensions, has afflicted the human species from the beginning. There is an ancient Egyptian hieroglyphic lament that lists the three greatest living hells in the following order: (1) to be in bed and sleep not; (2) to want the one who comes not; and (3) to try to please and please not.

In our own stress-ridden world, with its constantly accelerating pace, its problems that cannot be solved but at best merely managed, insomnia is more prevalent than ever. Our nightly journey into the world of sleep is often beset by as many difficulties and delays as a commuter train. Relaxation in general is at a premium, and new ways to achieve it are regularly offered to an anxious public. The fact that meditation, bio-feedback and other approaches to serenity are so popular only points up the fact that sleep—the most natural way to relax—is often hard to come by. A 1973 study made in Los Angeles showed, for instance, that 32 percent of the population suffered from some type of insomnia. And it is estimated that more than thirty million people in the United States are troubled by severe sleep problems.

There are three general types of insomnia. First, there is the inability to fall asleep, called *sleep-onset insomnia*. The individual may lie awake for hours reviewing the events of the day, ruminating endlessly about what should have been said or done, or worrying about what tomorrow will bring. Others have trouble falling asleep because they fear sleep— for a variety of reasons that will be explored more fully later in this chapter.

A second general type of insomnia, the inability to remain asleep, is most common of all, affecting 50 percent of insomniacs. The person suffering from this form will often have many wakenings during the night, of varying duration. In their experience of the sleep world it is as though they were traveling on a shuttle that takes them endlessly back and forth between the sleep world and the day world. This *sleep-maintenance insomnia* causes a fragmentation of the sleep experience and allows no profound rest.

Early morning awakening—*terminal insomnia*—constitutes a third type. The sufferer will awaken at an early morning hour, five or six o'clock, and be unable to get back to sleep. The French author Jean Dutourd wrote a novel, called *Five A.M.*, that focused entirely on the thoughts and feelings of a man who was the victim of this kind of insomnia. Such people tend to have more REM periods than the normal sleeper, bringing them to the verge of wakefulness many times in the course of the night. They often show a need to get back into the day world in order to bring their unsolved problems and anxieties under control. It seems likely, in fact, that many of those who claim to need only four or five hours of sleep a night are merely putting forth a positive interpretation of this kind of insomnia.

It is important to remember, however, that different people require differing amounts of sleep. Physical makeup as well as personality type are reflected in the sleep needs of the particular person. If you sleep only five or six hours a night, but feel alert and energetic during your waking hours, you are getting the sleep necessary to proper functioning and should not concern yourself with the fact that most people sleep seven or eight hours a night. Too often people persuade themselves that they are insomniacs on the basis of how much sleep other people—parents, friends, partners—appear to need.

Among those who do suffer from distinct sleep problems, some find them more upsetting than others. Studies have shown that younger males are the least likely to complain about their insomnia, while people over sixty who are having these difficulties most commonly find them disturbing enough to consult their physicians. In this older group, insomnia is sexist and affects more women than men. Retirement not only robs many older people of occupational identity and status, but of sleep as well. Worries about health and reduced income make it difficult to achieve the security necessary to sleep. Also, since sleep takes the individual out of the day world into an unknown new world each night, many older people become acutely aware of the "death-like" aspects of the sleep universe, and resist letting go of the reassuringly familiar surroundings of waking existence. Their fears are summed up in Shelley's line, "Till death like sleep might steal on me." There also may be physiological changes in older people that make it difficult for them to sleep soundly, and which add to any psychological problems of adjustment that they have.

Emotional stresses at any age can cause depression and

anxiety, leading to sleep difficulties. About 75 to 80 percent of those with psychological conflicts also suffer from some degree of sleep disturbance. Individuals in an anxiety state may desperately wish to escape into sleep—but because of their emotional tension are often unable to relax sufficiently for the normal sleep-enabling processes of the twilight zone to take hold. When a troubled person wants to sleep but cannot, it only intensifies the frightening feeling of being helpless in a world of peril.

Sexual problems can also cause insomnia in various ways. If an individual's twilight zone routine usually involves or follows sexual activity, then any problems involving sex will interfere with the established sleep pattern. Also, there are those who fear being overwhelmed by their sexual arousal, and thus resist the sleep world because of its close association with sex. They are afraid that they won't be able to control their sexual impulses in sleep; some are so insecure that they won't let anyone else sleep in the same room, for fear of being seduced.

Quite aside from such specific psychological disturbances, though, most of us suffer from transient episodes of insomnia at one time or another, during periods of specific stress. Job and financial pressures, marital difficulties, separation from a partner, divorce, the sickness or death of a loved one—any of the ills that we are heir to can cause sleeplessness. Such sleep disturbances are highly individualized, and may last only a few nights or at most several weeks, until the stress is relieved.

In our technological age, one well-known cause of transient insomnia is the upsetting of the biological clock that takes place when we jet from one time zone to another. The biological clock syndrome has more serious, long-term effects on people who work the night shift. While the rest of the world sleeps, thousands of men and women in the various service areas—transportation, communications, health, law enforcement and fire-fighting—are called upon to maintain essential around-the-clock functions. It has been estimated that 20 percent of the total working population live according to an inverted work-sleep pattern, working by night and sleeping by day. Such shift work is becoming increasingly common worldwide as industrial technology grows.

Night shift employees average only four to six hours of sleep on work days, creating a "sleep debt" that they try to repay by sleeping nine to fourteen hours on the weekend. Typically, the shift worker awakens more often and for longer periods during the daylight hours devoted to sleep than does the average person who sleeps at night. The problem is compounded, of course, when economic need or emergency situations result in the shift worker putting in overtime or doubling up on shifts. Because a shift worker sleeps fewer hours during the work week, and has more awakenings in the course of sleep, there is a tendency to develop a characteristic syndrome of tiredness, restlessness and irritability during his or her waking hours.

Prominent among the unwilling legions of the sleepless are those who suffer from such physical illnesses as arthritis and skeletal disorders, heart and circulatory disease, respiratory or neurological disturbances, and many other ailments. Their physical discomfort and the depression they feel concerning their health place them in double jeopardy, and they are all too easily conscripted into the insomniac ranks. A man lying in a hospital bed with his fractured leg suspended in traction before him is inevitably forced to focus exclusively on the broken leg. He thus cannot escape the depressing reality of his situation. Not only is the limb fractured, but indeed his entire existence: movement is halted and his freedom of behavior is held in suspension like the leg that confronts him hanging from the frame around his bed.

Insomnia is considered to be chronic only when it has lasted longer than three months. Whether the insomnia is transient or chronic, however, most people deal with it in the same way: they reach for the pill bottle. This "remedy" is often nothing of the kind, but merely makes for new and more serious sleep disturbances. The development of sleeping pill addiction through incorrect management of transient insomnia remains one of the large problems of medical practice. Self-medication with over-the-counter drugs in cases of temporary insomnia also carries distinct dangers. To get only a few hours' sleep for a few nights won't do you any real harm. You may operate with slightly diminished efficiency during the day, but that is not of major consequence. Temporary periods of insomnia, caused by specific life stresses, usually resolve themselves, but if you get hooked on pills this transient insomnia can become chronic.

Two thirds of those suffering from significant sleep disturbances take their problems to a physician. Treatment of these twenty million patients usually focuses upon the immediate relief of the patient's sleeplessness. Thus the real causes of the sleep disturbance may not be adequately identified, and insight into the relation between the symptom and possible medical, psychological, or situational problems is not likely to be attained. The sleep world is a natural human habitat, and when people find that they are not at home in the night universe, the cause of their difficulty almost invariably lies in the *day* world. If the tendency is to focus on the symptom and merely to prescribe hypnotics (sleeping medication), there can be unfortunate complications.

There is an enormous overuse of both prescription and

nonprescription sleeping pills. This abuse is exacerbated by the fact that—with one or two important exceptions—most such drugs become ineffective after two weeks because of the patient's increasing tolerance to them. Most over-the-counter sleep medications are not effective in the dosages used in the pills. Yet, if used in larger doses, these biologically powerful drugs can be dangerous. Barbiturates, available only by prescription, are effective for short periods, but over a longer time can become highly addictive physically. There are some newer drugs that do not have this drawback, and which have made obsolete the use of barbiturates for chronic insomnia. They may, however, cause a psychological dependency, and they alleviate the symptoms without dealing with the underlying cause of the insomnia.

Once the individual develops a tolerance for the drug he is taking—and it ceases to be effective in the usual dosage—it is common to start increasing the number of pills taken. Yet patients using drugs chronically (longer than six months) still have much difficulty in falling asleep and staying asleep. Once their tolerance develops, the pill won't work. In ordinary insomnia, preceding the use of drugs, the duration of the REM phases remains the same, but there is less slow wave sleep. With chronic drug use, there is a marked *decrease* in REM sleep, and a variety of wave disturbances occurs during the other stages. In other words, the patient is worse off than ever in terms of getting a satisfactory night's sleep.

In addition, a drug-withdrawal syndrome often sets in. The body automatically tries to fight off the effects of the alien drug. Resistance to the drug keeps pace with the amount being taken, so that both the amount of medication in the body and the resistance to it steadily climb to higher levels. As a result, even though a person takes a considerable dosage before going to sleep, the effects of the drug may wear off in the middle of the night. At this point, a phenomenon called *REM rebound* occurs. With REM rebound there is a massive increase in dreaming, as though the lid had been lifted on Pandora's box. These dreams may show a frightening, nightmarish quality and, as might be expected, cause repeated awakenings during the night.

When patients who find that their sleep medication is less and less effective try to stop taking the drug, the result is often a drug-withdrawal insomnia with nightmarish awakenings. This problem is complicated by psychological worries about the ability to get along without the drug, and by a general nervousness and agitation.

In order to avoid drug-withdrawal insomnia, a chronically used sleep medication should be decreased only at the rate of one dosage per week. Thus, if a person has been taking a hypnotic each night, it will take at least seven weeks to complete withdrawal from the sleeping medication.

Clearly, then, drugs are not a satisfactory answer to insomnia in a great many cases. When transient insomnia caused by temporary life stresses is mishandled, the vicious circle outlined above can all too easily be set in motion. But is there nothing else that can be done to help mild or transient insomnia? How might the problem be eased without using drugs? Are there natural techniques—derived from an understanding of sleep positions, from the concept of the twilight zone and the nature of the sleep world itself—that could be used instead?

The first key to good sound sleep is to remember the importance of the twilight zone as a period of decompression. Entering the sleep world might be compared to landing an airplane. A plane flying at 30,000 feet can't be brought to earth successfully all at one go. Speed must be decreased, altitude gradually lowered, the wheels locked into place and the wing flaps adjusted. As we saw in Chapter One, the human body cannot make the transition from the day world to the sleep world at full speed either. If we return home from a full day's work and an evening on the town, having been on the go for as much as sixteen hours, and simply throw off our clothes and get into bed, sleep is likely to be difficult to achieve because of our aroused state.

It has been said that sleep cannot be captured by force, but must be wooed like a lover. The folk-wisdom of many countries and cultures has addressed itself to the question of how this courtship might best be conducted. Some of these folk techniques are amusingly bizarre, but the majority make a great deal of sense. And it is interesting to note how many of them seem intuitively to grasp the principles of the twilight zone process—even though they predate current scientific knowledge concerning sleep by generations.

Throughout history there has been a great emphasis placed on what one should (or should not) eat and drink shortly before bedtime if one wishes to sleep well. The matter of food digestion is a major one. The actual process of human digestion was first studied scientifically by an American frontier physician named Beaumont in a classic case involving the treatment of an Indian with a gunshot wound of the abdomen. The wound created a kind of flap or pouch—like a kangaroo's—that gave Beaumont a direct view into the Indian's stomach. By observing the digestive processes, he made a number of discoveries. Among other things, he compiled a table listing the periods of time it took for various foods to be digested. The following are a few examples from "Beaumont's Table":

Fresh eggs whipped,
*   fresh salmon trout broiled*
*   or fried,*
*   venison steak broiled*   — 1½ hours to digest
Roast suckling pig   — 2½ hours
Domesticated turkey   — 2½ hours/15 mins

It is amusing to note that wild turkey, a tougher bird, takes three minutes longer than the domesticated variety to be digested.

In general, therefore, if you allow two and a half hours between eating and retiring for the night, the stomach will most likely have completed its digestive task. Of course, if you insist upon a plate of chili, a hot curry, or a multitude of mushrooms, you are likely to suffer from certain gastric reverberations even after these foods have been digested. They may produce acidity, gas distension and cramps, bringing about repeated awakenings during the night.

Recently, however, it has been discovered that some kinds of food contain a chemical called L-tryptophan, which facilitates sleep. It is found in such protein-rich foods as meat, cheese and eggs. The best source of L-tryptophan is turkey (presumably either wild or domesticated), which may be one reason why we tend to fall asleep so easily after Thanksgiving dinner. One gram of L-tryptophan cuts down the time it takes to fall asleep by half. Thus, if one must eat shortly before sleeping, a light snack rich in protein will help induce sleep and counterbalance the lack of time for complete digestion.

What is the relationship between drink and sleep? This is a question that has been much discussed down through the ages. In Aubrey's *Brief Lives* it is reported that Francis Bacon, the great Elizabethan philosopher, often drank "a good draught of strong Beer . . . to-bedwards, to lay his working Fancy asleep, which otherwise would keep him from sleeping a great part of the night." To this day, alcohol remains a greatly favored hypnotic for those who have difficulty sleeping. While small doses of alcohol have a sedative effect on the higher levels of the nervous system, heavy use of alcohol results in the suppression of the REM phases, fragmentation of sleep, and the distressing REM-rebound phenomenon discussed in respect to sleeping pill abuse, so that there is no consistent rest. In cases of acute alcohol abuse, such as a prolonged drinking bout, it takes six weeks—after abstinence and detoxification—for fully normal sleep patterns without fragmentation, to be reestablished.

Many other potions have been recommended at various times as sleep inducers. The English were particularly fond of bedtime "possets," a kind of punch, and concocted hundreds of recipes for them from the seventeenth century on. Most of these possets were laced with alcohol—whether wine, ale or brandy—but the base was usually a combination of eggs and milk. The amount of alcohol was modest, and, as we now know, the presence of L-tryptophan in milk and eggs does aid sleep. It seems likely, in fact, that these possets were probably as effective as most present-day sleeping pills, especially the over-the-counter variety. For the insomniac with a culinary bent, the following recipe from T. Dawson's *The Widdowe's Treasure* (1595) is offered:

> First take the Milke and seethe it on the fire, and before it seethe, put in your Egges according to the quantity of your Milke, but see that your egges be tempered with some of your milke that standeth on the fire; and you must stir until it seethe, and beginneth to rise, then take it from the fire, and have your drink ready on a chafing dish of coales, and put your milke into the bason as it standeth, and

cover it, and let it stand awile, then take it up, and cast on Ginger and Cinamon.

The "drink" mentioned in this recipe would probably have been sack; the experts are divided on exactly what sack was, but it appears to have been a member of the sherry family. Since this posset resembles a kind of eggnog, rum would seem the sensible modern-day substitute.

A less exotic and less harmful potion would be a plain glass of milk, preferably warm. Milk not only contains L-tryptophan, but is for many people a drink that revives childhood feelings of security. Chamomile tea also seems to be a good hypnotic. Drinks containing caffeine generally have the opposite effect from what is desired. However, when sleeplessness is caused by restless overfatigue, a cup of coffee or tea will often aid sleep by eliminating the sleep-inhibiting fatigue. Tea has half as much caffeine as coffee, and most colas have about a third as much.

With the stomach satisfied, the comfort of the rest of the body must be assured. Once in bed, the proper degree of warmth is important. As was pointed out in the first chapter, a certain degree of coolness is conducive to sleep. If we are too cold—or too hot—though, sleep will be more difficult to achieve. Nevertheless, some folk remedies for insomnia do suggest exposing oneself to various degrees of heat and cold. The warm bath is much recommended, in that it relaxes the muscles and eases nervous tension. At the other extreme is the suggestion that one strip naked and stand in front of an open window until one begins to shiver, and then jump immediately into a bed that has been warmed with a hot water bottle. This "reverse sauna" approach is clearly only for those with polar bear constitutions.

In the popular literature on sleep, a great deal of attention is paid to the feet. In part, it may be because the feet do much work in the day world that they are singled out for special concern at bedtime. More importantly, they are among the body's major temperature regulators. Cold feet are regarded as a particularly vexing problem. Icy feet, quite aside from keeping their possessor awake, can be equally disturbing to a sleep partner, and a definite deterrent to sleep-world intimacy. "Never go to bed with cold feet, or cold heart," wrote William Hone in 1841. Obviously, in couple sleep, the former might easily lead to the latter.

Russian nobles used to have the soles and heels of their feet scratched by their servants in order to facilitate sleep. This technique, like a good massage, could be used by a sleep partner—provided the partner is willing and the insomniac not ticklish. In the past a lengthy brushing of the hair before retiring was regarded as an excellent soporific for women, but the additional, cosmetic advantages of this procedure have been nullified by the ubiquitous hair dryer with brush attachment, whose electronic buzz is hardly suited for the twilight zone but rather effective at goading the individual back into the day world in the morning.

Various cultures have special techniques for putting their children to sleep. Korean mothers scratch their babies gently on the stomach in order to calm and soothe them. Spanish women often stroke the child's upper spine. Some Mediterranean mothers will rub the genitals of a fretful male child. All of these tactile reassurances reflect once again, in embryonic form, the ancient association between sleep and sex.

Once the individual is in bed, the matter of the best position for entry into the sleep world becomes paramount. Down through the ages, virtually every conceivable basic sleep position has been recommended at some point as *the* best one in which to sleep—only to be repudiated by some other commentator. Some of these suggestions are particularly fetching. In *Natural and Artificial Directions for Health,* published in 1602, William Vaughn suggests: "Sleep first on your right side with your mouth open, and let your night cappe have a hole in the top, through which the vapour may go out." Even earlier, in 1589, one Thomas Cogan wrote: ". . . to lye on either side, is good. But to lye upright upon the backe, or groveling upon the bellie is unwholesome." Some commentators say that to lie on the left side is bad for the heart—while others insist that it is good. And so it goes.

All of these categorical pronouncements were of course made in ignorance of the fact that our sleep positions are determined by the essential way we live in the world. There is no such thing as a sleep position that is best for everyone. We all will assume the positions—both an alpha position and an omega position—that give us the security we need to go to sleep and stay asleep. The sleep world is a private one, and though it is governed by certain fundamental physiological conditions, the final arbiter of the sleep world is the individual himself.

There are, however, two yoga positions, outlined by Harvey Day in his book *About Yoga,* that closely approximate the basic sleep positions chosen by many people, and thus bear quoting here. The first parallels the royal position.

> Lie on your back on a firm, flat bed, without a pillow. Close your eyes and relax your limbs utterly. This is not easy. Take each part of your body in turn: eyes, mouth, chin, tongue, neck, arms, hands, stomach, thighs, legs, feet, toes. Then start again and go through the entire list. Imagine that you are sinking right through the bed. You may have to relax each organ or limb a number of times before complete relaxation is achieved, though the possibility is that you will fall asleep without quite knowing when or how.

The relaxation technique outlined here is very similar to those suggested by a number of writers who, in recent books on relaxation and related approaches to tranquillity, have drawn upon yoga techniques. Another position outlined by Day recalls the Hero position discussed in Chapter Five.

> Use a soft, low pillow and place the head firmly on it, giving the neck no strain and no work to do. Sleep on the right side with the legs straight down the bed, but not stiff. Place the left leg over and along it, with the left foot either slightly overlapping the right, or behind it. The left arm, with the palm facing down, lies along the body and the thigh: the right arm slightly in front of the body. If no pillow is used, the right arm may be folded and the right arm—wrist and hand—placed under the head.
> Once mastered, this position brings sound, restful sleep.

As an alternative approach, a more direct technique called "Swedish Massage" can be used. A two-foot-long piece of broomstick (or dowel) is placed beneath the spine as one lies on one's back. (A rubber ball may also be used.) At first you will be extremely aware of the stick or ball; the only way to make yourself comfortable is to thoroughly relax the muscles in the area of the object. Once you have relaxed sufficiently so that the presence of the dowel is comfortable and virtually unnoticeable, it should be moved a few inches farther up toward the middle of the back. By the time it has been moved up to the base of the neck, you should be fully relaxed. I believe that this technique is related to the use of the Japanese wooden pillow, and of the wooden headrests common among several ancient cultures, including the Sumerian and the Egyptian. With such a hard object beneath the head, comfort can be achieved only through profound muscular relaxation—which would automatically induce the alpha state that heralds the beginning of sleep.

In addition to muscular relaxation, it is also necessary to

avoid distracting thoughts and day world concerns. Again, the suggestions made over the centuries on how to manage this withdrawal from the day world are legion. Reading has always been much recommended, but the question of whether to read a dull book or an interesting one invariably arises. This seems to be an entirely personal matter—a good thriller may take one person so completely out of his own world that he immediately becomes drowsy, while the same book will stimulate another reader to tingling arousal. Orson Welles claims to peruse the *History of MacHenry County, Ill.*, while others opt for old *Congressional Records* or the works of almost any philosopher.

Those who find reading too arousing often prefer to "count sheep" or use similar repetitive mental exercises. The composing of limericks or, especially, the use of anagrams works for some people, preventing them from thinking about the fact that the car needs repairing, that their in-laws are due for a visit, or whatever other day world trial awaits them. For instance, one can put together the letters of the alphabet in a sequence based on the vowels—as in bab, cab, dab, fab, followed eventually by beb, bec, bed, bef, until one gets to zuz.

Others find such techniques unavailing, and prefer more abstract perceptions. They may focus on an imaginary far pinpoint of light, or conceive of a dark ball rolling toward them from a great distance, getting larger and larger until it absorbs them. I personally prefer to imagine a gray-black wall, covering the entire visual field, on which a circle is drawn round and round in a counterclockwise direction. If one is left-handed, the figure should be drawn clockwise. This induces some degree of thought strain, so that the attention is diverted from the day's activities and focused instead on a monotonous, repetitive activity that has certain lulling elements, a rising and falling, involved in it.

The way we breathe, and the rate of respiration, are extremely important in achieving bodily relaxation. As we have seen, in sleep itself the rate of respiration is slowed. People who are able to regulate their breathing, through the use of yoga or other methods, have an advantage in terms of falling asleep. If the rate of respiration is slowed, other bodily processes, particularly the heartbeat, will follow suit. Breathing through the nose with the mouth closed, exhaling with moderate force, is conducive to achieving the breathing pattern typical of sleep. Singers, who are taught to breathe from the diaphragm in order to be able to support their voices more fully, are usually very sound sleepers.

People who have difficulty breathing are particularly likely to have problems sleeping. The asthmatic often finds it necessary to sleep upright, or with several pillows under the head. Sleep *apnea* is a fairly rare, but often overlooked, cause of insomnia; the person suffering from this disability stops breathing for a moment, and then starts again with a kind of snort. The decrease in oxygen intake caused by this disorder can lead to constant choking awakenings in the course of the night.

As we pass through the twilight zone, it is necessary to achieve muscular relaxation, a quiescent stomach, the banishment of day world thoughts, and proper breathing. A number of other general principles should be remembered, as well.

First, a regular sleep pattern should be established. As we have seen, our biological clocks are easily thrown out of kilter. People whose life-styles are irregular, and who may go to bed at eleven o'clock one night but at three in the morning the next, are likely to encounter sleep problems. Those who go to bed at varying times often do not allow for the proper period of repose before attempting to sleep, aggravating the difficulties still further.

Full twilight zone relaxation requires darkness and the absence of noise—in spite of those few individuals who prefer to sleep with the radio playing or who may fall asleep in a lighted room or even with their eyes open. Studies have shown, in fact, that people whose bedrooms are decorated in vibrant color schemes have greater difficulty in getting to sleep.

Many external noises cannot be completely shut out, of course. But most people are selective about what they hear in the night, and will not be disturbed by normal sounds that they have grown used to. People who find themselves waking at a certain time in the middle of the night, time and time again, are often responding to some external stimulus of which they are unaware. One woman, who found that she was waking each night at 2:20 A.M., went to a doctor for help. Instead of prescribing sleeping pills, the doctor suggested that she set her alarm clock for 2:15, in order to discover if there might be some unusual sound that was waking her. She found, in fact, that her next-door neighbor, who worked a shift beginning at 3:00 A.M., was letting his screen door slam as he left the house. Once the woman knew the cause of her awakenings, the noise ceased to disturb her.

If all else fails, and a person cannot fall asleep—or wakes and cannot get back to sleep—it is better to get up and read, write letters, make out shopping lists than to lie in the darkness desperately seeking sleep that will not come. Indeed, after fifteen minutes to half an hour of such activity, many people find themselves feeling sleepy. Their tensions have been relieved by focusing on something other than the vexation of their insomnia, and it is often possible to fall quickly asleep.

Beyond these general principles, however, I have evolved a method of treating mild to moderate insomnia that makes specific use of the knowledge that there is an alpha (or relaxation) sleep position, as well as a characterological omega position that is adopted in full sleep. The individual should make use of whatever muscular relaxation techniques seem to work best to facilitate passage through the twilight zone. Slow, regular nasal breathing is also recommended. One or more of the various repetitive mental exercises mentioned may prove helpful in banishing intrusive day world thoughts. But in addition to these devices, the reader's knowledge of his or her own sleep positions should be put to work.

Begin by assuming your habitual alpha relaxation position —whether lying on the back, the side, or prone. Awareness of two paradoxical sensations should be cultivated. To begin with, the body will seem to be weighing more heavily on the bed. One should also feel a certain lightening of the self, as though one were floating. Some people who suffer from insomnia find this duality of sensation disturbing—they are resisting the sleep world. Instead, one should let oneself enter fully into the experiencing of these two reciprocal sensations, feeling the floating sensation more completely one moment, the growing heaviness of the body the next. When these two characteristic elements of sleep onset are allowed to coexist, each will enhance the other. As this process is taking place, it is important to continue breathing through the nose, exhaling with mild force, as described earlier.

Gradually, the floating sensation will come to predominate. When one feels that one wants only to continue floating, the edge of sleep has been reached. Now, one should turn immediately into one's accustomed omega or characterological position—the position in which the individual usually prefers to spend most of the night. And the sleep world will have been entered.

The normal time it takes to fall asleep is approximately fifteen minutes. If one's attempts to achieve sleep have been in vain after that length of time, it can be helpful to use the omega position even so. Since the omega position is most deeply associated with sleep itself, it can sometimes have a more relaxing effect than the usual alpha position, when there are difficulties in going to sleep. But the change from an alpha to an omega position is a natural progression, and in many cases the answer to the insomnia problem is to assume a new, more effective alpha position.

I have previously noted several cases in which patients assumed a different twilight zone alpha position when they were going through a particularly anxious period in their lives. Most of us have such "fall-back" positions. A person may on occasion find that it is necessary to lie prone in order to achieve the preliminary security required for sleep, even though his usual alpha position is semi-fetal. Or a semi-fetal sleeper may adopt a full-fetal alpha position when under stress. By developing your awareness of the positions in which you sleep, by knowing their significance and the degrees of security or insecurity that they reflect, it can become possible for you to *choose* the alpha or omega sleep position that in fact most fully epitomizes your security-insuring behavior at a given time. As has been noted many times in previous chapters, people do change their sleep positions when they encounter particular stresses, or when they feel especially relaxed and can let go of certain defenses. By becoming aware of such changes, and of their significance, a position appropriate to the way one feels can be assumed in combating insomnia.

If you are going through a period of stress, but assume your usual alpha relaxation position nevertheless, then the position in which you are trying to enter the sleep world will not be in concert with your life at that moment. In time, if the stress continues, an individual will inevitably change his sleep position, bringing the body in the dark into line with the way he is living in the waking world. But it may take a period of time before that transition is complete. If, through his knowledge of the meanings of the various sleep positions, he is able to adopt a new position, on a temporary basis, that is in proper symmetry with his fundamental day patterns of existence, he will in many cases be able to fall asleep more easily. The stress and anxiety may still be present, but because they are being dealt with by means of the chosen sleep position, a reduction of insomnia and easier entry into the sleep world can be achieved.

CHAPTER

EARLY WARNING SIGNS—
SLEEP-POSITION ANALYSIS

"Our little life is rounded in a sleep," says Prospero in *The Tempest.*

In a state markedly similar to the REM phase, the fetus sleeps in the womb. The newborn infant sleeps about seventeen hours per day in its cradle. The child seeks out the changing sleep positions that reflect the stages of the developing self. The teenager and the young adult display their full individuality in the sleep world, choosing the characterological positions that delineate the ways they will live their lives. Couple partners attune their sleep posture to one another, making explicit in the night world their dyadic relationship. Troubled individuals express their conflicts in the clear night language of the body. Our loves, fears and hates, our feelings about ourselves and our world, even our physical frailties—all the sagas of our lives are evoked in the dark as we pass through the years toward the ultimate sleep.

At every point along the way, our knowledge of the special dimensions and experiences of the sleep universe, and our understanding of the significance of sleep positions, can help us to discover ourselves more fully. Our sleep world is full of signs and signals that indicate the directions our lives are taking.

* * *

The parent looking in on a sleeping child may often be surprised to see the small form folded into some awkward or peculiar position. The child may be sleeping on its knees, back raised, in the Sphinx position. Or the Switch position may be assumed, with the body rebelliously reversed in the bed. Keeping in mind the plasticity of the growing child, and the continuing evolution of sleep positions as described in Chapter Four, the parent may merely smile, settle the diminutive sleeping being in a more normal position, and close the door again. The temporary adoption of a strange sleep position is really nothing to cause special concern—to realize that fact can save the parent needless worry.

On the other hand, if a child is found to be sleeping in a single unusual position over a period of weeks or months, a significant disturbance may be indicated. By observing the position, it is possible to gain some insight into the nature of the child's problems on the basis of the meanings that sleep-position analysis will yield. With such knowledge, parents and pediatricians—as well as nurses, school guidance counselors, and social workers—can more directly grasp what is going on in the child's life. Since children are sometimes guarded about what is bothering them, sleep-position analysis allows parents and others to recognize the existence and meaning of problems when the child is unwilling or unable to put them into words.

By the late teens, sleep positions are fairly well defined for the individual. Thus, an exotic position adopted at this age can carry considerable significance. When such a position occurs in combination with unusual or symptomatic waking behavior, the need for professional consultation may be indicated. A young person encountering severe adjustment difficulties in school or college, or who seems to be having trouble in the area of adult social, sexual and work relations, will give expression to these problems in the sleep world, sometimes revealing in this way the key to a conflict that has not been mastered.

As young adults begin to seek out compatible partners in their twenties, a new application of the knowledge of sleep positions comes into play. For example, a young woman who is a patient of mine went on a vacation to the Caribbean. Despite the fact that she had just recently broken off a relationship with a man, and was somewhat wary of entering into a new one, she had an affair with a fellow vacationer, a Frenchman, while she was away. On her return, she reported that she thought she was in love with the Frenchman, and was debating the possible risks and rewards of trying to continue their romance. The fact that he was now back in France, while she was in New York, was clearly a formidable obstacle, but one she was willing to try to deal with. Nevertheless, there was something else that bothered her about the relationship—on all but two occasions, the man had immediately turned his back to her and gone to sleep after they had made love.

In the course of therapy, I had discussed her own and her previous lover's sleep positions with her, and she was aware, in a general way, of the significance of sleep positions and of the fact that they reveal feelings and a person's characteristic behavior patterns. She said that on the first night of her holiday with the Frenchman, he had gone to sleep facing her and holding her. But on subsequent nights, he had turned his back on her almost the moment they finished making love and retreated to his own side of the bed. She had asked him if he was aware of doing this, and he replied that a girl friend he had in Paris had complained about the same thing. Even though he was aware that his sleep-world behavior distressed women, he was basically unable to change it, for it was fundamental to the way he lived. Thus, he continued to turn his back until their last night together, when anticipation of separation, with its attendant pangs, caused him again to sleep facing her, to reassure himself against her imminent disappearance.

The young woman was caught between conflicting feelings about the Frenchman—should she or shouldn't she try to continue the relationship? Would it eventually go anywhere? She decided that the chances of trying to continue a long-distance romance with him were limited. Since the man had difficulty in relating to her in an open face-to-face way when they were occupying the same bed, it seemed unlikely that over the long run he would be able to respond fully to her genuine feelings for him, especially with the added problem of an ocean between them. In his sleep position, he had indicated that there already existed a gulf between them in the sleep world; the difficulties would only be compounded by the geographic distance between them in the post-vacation day world.

The young woman's application of her knowledge about sleep positions can similarly be put to use in many tentative couple relationships. When one is sufficiently attracted to someone to contemplate entering into a long-term relationship—that might possibly lead to marriage—a host of factors are always more or less taken into account. We form our opinions of people, and come to know and understand them, on the basis of both large and small aspects of their personalities and their behavior toward us and others. A woman who likes a man very much, but finds some fault with his life-style, may have second thoughts about how deeply she wants to become involved with him. We make up our minds about our compatibility with people in large part on the basis of physical attractiveness, personality fit, social attributes and mutual interests. But now, the reader of this book has a further important clue to consider in evaluating the viability of a couple relationship—how one's contemplated long-term partner sleeps. Obviously, the person's sleep behavior is most often made known, in today's world, through the direct experience of spending the night together. But people usually find the concept of sleep positions interesting enough to discuss their habits even when the relationship has not progressed to the point of sexual intimacy.

The young woman who had the vacation affair liked most things about her Frenchman—his sensitive intelligence, his charm, the tender and skillful way he made love. But what she did not like was the way he ended up shutting her out of his sleep world. Rightly, she felt that if he was going to shut her out there, he probably would shut her out of other important parts of his life. She felt that in the long run no amount of intelligence, charm and good sex could substitute for the complete openness and mutual warmth she wanted in a serious ongoing relationship. That was the most vital requirement, and the way he slept indicated that it was lacking. Because she did enjoy his company very much, she continued to see him, but on a realistic basis, recognizing that it was a limited relationship. Because she had no false hopes, she avoided the fruitless yearning and pining after a man she knew could never completely satisfy her needs.

The way we sleep is the way we live. If we are made uncomfortable by the way a partner sleeps—whether that person withdraws from us in sleep, or insensitively tries to smother us when we sometimes want to retreat within our own life-space; whether frustrating us by curling up out of reach in a corner of the bed, or by dominating three quarters of the bed-space with outstretched limbs—we are likely to find ourselves uncomfortable with the expression of these same tendencies in other phases of the person's life. If we are strongly disturbed by the way someone relates to us in sleep, then—whatever the individual's other virtues—we have a basic indication that we are not going to like the way that person relates to us by day either, once the "honeymoon" is over.

To ignore the way a person sleeps, because we like other things about them, is to pass up an important clue to that person's fundamental nature. No partner in a couple relationship likes everything about the other. But while it is possible to accept many kinds of minor habits, idiosyncracies and lapses in a loved one, and to make a long-term relationship work in spite of these, it is difficult to overlook a person's most intrinsic patterns of being. By observing their sleep positions, one can discern the essential ways they feel and behave in their world, and how they relate to the important people in it—an incisive outline that is free from the blurring distractions of everyday life. This understanding gives added depth to one person's perception of how the other would fit into the life they might share together.

Couples who have been together for some time can also make use of their knowledge of sleep positions to keep their fingers on the pulse of their emotional union. Changes in the sleep position of a partner can, as we have seen, indicate what is currently happening in the partner's life-space. A sudden or dramatic change should be taken seriously. When a couple habitually sleep in the Spoon position, and one partner abruptly abandons this intimate posture to sleep on the far edge of the bed with a turned back, trouble is almost certainly brewing. Being aware of the significance of such changes can sometimes make it possible for a couple to focus on and deal with a conflict before it becomes too disruptive. In addition, since sleep positions so clearly reveal the pattern of the couple relationship as a whole, partners can gain insight into their shared lives and arrive at a fuller understanding of one another's important emotional needs. A disturbed form of sleep behavior—such as the husband who nightly began sidling out of bed like a crab—can indicate a marital rift serious enough to require professional help.

For individuals whose problems lead them at some point in their lives to enter psychotherapy, sleep-position analysis can have a special importance, both to the patient and to the therapist. There are very few indicators by which a therapist can overtly demonstrate the behavioral and personality changes taking place in patients during therapy—in their way of life and in their feelings about themselves and their world. Sleep positions have the potential of offering "hard" evidence that the therapy is having specific effects and following an expected course. It adds to the usual means of making such estimations of progress and growth. The night language of the body provides a finely calibrated instrument by which to measure the degree and direction of the psychological growth of the individual in treatment.

Several cases have already been presented that show how strikingly sleep positions impart an individual's capacity for intimacy. A particularly clear example is provided by the young man discussed in Chapter Seven, who at the beginning of therapy slept in a full-fetal position with his back to his partner, but who eventually evolved to the point of sleeping on his back and took pleasure in having his partner rest her head on his chest.

Another case, in which a dramatic change recently took place after years in treatment, involves a woman in her late thirties. At the beginning of treatment, she had to be hospitalized briefly because of severe depression; she had just been rejected by a partner and her fragile personality was badly shaken. Both her sexual and loving responsiveness had long been under the sway of inhibitions caused by a turbulent, destructive family history. During her lengthy treatment, she had a number of alliances of relatively long duration, but they were stormy.

Almost a year ago, she succeeded in breaking off a relationship in which she had allowed herself to be heavily exploited, a price she paid for the security of having a partner. Overcoming her depression at breaking-up, she established herself more independently, living by herself while she worked more intensively to come to grips with the genesis and expression of her emotional difficulties. In recent months, the sense of freedom, stability and self-growth has begun to be very evident. Since the end of her last relationship, she had had no others, until, by happy accident she met a man in his fifties at a New Year's Eve party and fell suddenly and profoundly in love. With this lover she achieved orgasm easily and with a completely fulfilling response—something that in her prior experience had been impossible.

This woman was basically a prone sleeper. When in a depressed state, she would sleep in a full-fetal position. In her relationship with her recent lover, she slept on her left side in the Spoon position with him. The man lay behind her, in close contact and embracing her with his arm. The protective father-figure implications are clear here, but although ambivalent and disturbing emotions concerning her father had played an important role in her life, their restrictive effects were now loosened in this relationship. During the course of the night, she and her lover would reverse position, and she would lie behind him, for she was now able to embrace a different kind of relationship with a man.

She reported that when she had slept with anyone previously, she and her partner would immediately turn their backs on one another upon going to sleep. Thus, her new-found ability to respond fully and easily to a love relationship was paralleled by concrete sleep-world evidence of her new potential for loving openness. Her couple sleep position now showed a new sense of herself. While her verbalizations in therapy concerning her growth were necessarily subjective, her changed couple sleep position gave clear testimony that she had truly opened new potentials of living for herself.

An understanding of sleep positions can also be useful in helping to spot developing physical illness. A woman acquaintance of mine was operated on for a tumor of her right auditory nerve; the tumor had developed to the point of causing deafness in the right ear. While casually discussing sleep positions with her at a party, she told me that she habitually slept in a semi-fetal position on the left side. In addition, she reported, for the past ten years she had been in the habit of putting her head between two pillows, with the upper pillow placed squarely over her right ear. It can be deduced—and she verified the deduction when asked—that the early growth of the hearing nerve tumor resulted in tinnitus (a ringing sensation) in her right ear. Ascribing this ringing to external stimuli, she had tried to eliminate it by placing the pillow over her ear, not realizing that in her case the tinnitus was an early sign of this type of tumor.

The interesting feature here is that the neurosurgeon had told her that the tumor had probably been developing for ten years! Thus the early development of the tumor presumably coincided with her use of the second pillow over the affected ear. Had medicine been aware of the messages communicated by sleep positions, it is possible that her change from a simple semi-fetal position to this striking variation on the Ostrich might have alerted physicians to the pathology taking place in her right auditory nerve. The existence of the tumor might well have been discovered years earlier, and been removed before it resulted in the complete loss of hearing in the right ear, or in other possibly more dangerous complications.

I have previously discussed sleeping positions in relation to heart cases. In other physical conditions, sleeping positions form part of the complex reaction of the individual to his pain or disability. Individuals with ulcers, stones in the kidneys, hernias, and other physical syndromes often change their sleep positions in order to diminish the painful pressure around tender or inflamed parts of the body. Here again, a change in sleep position that is connected with the guarding or easing of a particular anatomical region can also be an early warning signal, indicating a situation that needs rapid attention. The clinical usefulness of seeking clues to medical problems in an individual's sleep position is readily apparent, further extending the range of insights that can be gained from a knowledge of our sleep world activity.

CHAPTER

BEING IN
THE NIGHT

THROUGHOUT OUR LIVES, in sickness and health, living alone or in a couple relationship, our sleep world behavior unfolds the story of our particular existence. It reflects every turn of the plot, every crisis, every change. In fact, as we have seen, our sleep world behavior sometimes reveals our true feelings about a situation or a relationship before we have even begun to face those feelings in the waking world.

In the twentieth century, our knowledge of the sleep world has expanded enormously. Freud's recognition and analysis of the meaning of dreams, Aserinsky and Kleitman's discoveries concerning the correlation between rapid eye movements and dreaming, the continuing work of many researchers on brain chemistry, hormonal activity and sleep dysfunction —all these important discoveries are like the pieces of a jigsaw puzzle that have not previously been assembled satisfactorily.

Over the past several years, as I came to understand the significance of sleep positions and the full dimensions of the sleep world, a whole new panorama of meaning gradually unfolded itself. The more I discovered about the ways in which we live in the sleep world, the more I learned about the night language of the body, the more profoundly revelatory the sleep experience showed itself to be. It is a rich world, this dark universe in which we spend on the average over twenty years of our lifetimes. It is unlike any other world of which we have knowledge, with its own special laws. The orientations that govern our waking lives are transformed in sleep. The dimensions of space and time are revealed in special ways in sleep consciousness. Our sense of ourselves expands to take in the myriad facets of our universe of experience. We can be a rock, an animal, another person—all in rapid succession. In the sleep world we partake richly of the vast possibilities of existence and of a sense of the cosmos.

Yet, remarkably, we inhabit this expanding, unbounded universe in ways that are unique to each one of us. No two individuals respond to or experience the sleep world in the same way. How we behave in the sleep world, what we dream, what we do with our bodies, reflect the intrinsic way that we live in the waking world. The concrete stage of our waking world, however, is limited—we can only be in one place at one time, in an apartment, on a train, sitting at an office desk. In the sleep world we can be in all these places and many more in an instant. Yet where we find ourselves in sleep, and how we react to being there, will always tell much about the particular people we are, awake or asleep.

We dream, and our special anticipations and perspectives are expressed in the kaleidoscopic events of those dreams. A person who dreams of a rock is showing the flinty character of his life at that time. A patient who had a dream image of steel girders was illustrating that her life consisted of rigidities, which supported her emotionally, but at the same time limited her spontaneity and flexibility. The third-century B.C. Chinese philosopher, Chuang-tzu, who dreamed that he was a butterfly "fluttering hither and thither," wakened to find that he was a man—but wondered if he might not really be a butterfly dreaming that he was a man. His butterfly dream elegantly expresses this philosopher's day world search for the nectar of truth.

But are we the rock, the girder, the butterfly? In our sleep we can be. And what we choose to be in the night world shows what we are as human beings. The night world and the day world are not mutually exclusive. The time that we spend in sleep is not merely a hiatus between one day and another. Experiments have shown the high accuracy and validity of sleep judgment and thinking. The sleep world is just as valid a state of being as the day world—we do not live in the sleep world in a state of suspension, we simply live in it differently. The special bodily and thinking experiences of this night world are as meaningful as those of waking life. The significance of our dreams has been long established; the acuity of sleep-thinking has been recognized. But our bodily occupation of the night world is equally telling. During the day we exist in both a thinking and a bodily way, and so too do we in the night. The full extent of our humanness is encompassed in the night world as it is in the light of day.

We lie upon our stomach, our side, our back. Our legs may be spread wide or tightly clenched, our arms extended or pulled in close about our body. And these positions in the darkness tell the true story of our changing lives, of how we feel about ourselves, our day world and the important people in it. In the night our bodies move toward or withdraw from our sleep partners in a vivid explication of our feelings about our husbands, wives and lovers.

The great paradox of the sleep world is that while we can be anything in it, can experience it in ways that are markedly different from the viewpoint of waking life, we nevertheless explore this universe, and situate ourselves in it according to our most fundamental personal needs and desires.

Throughout the whole course of our human existence, from birth to death, we sleep as we live, and in our sleep world we attune ourselves to our waking experience, to all of our enduring history, to all of our ongoing quests.